OXFORD MEDICAL PUBLICATIONS

The Maudsley Handbook of Practical Psychiatry

Sixth edition

T0177608

The Maudsley Handbook of Practical Psychiatry

Sixth edition

Edited by

Gareth Owen

Clinical Senior Lecturer
Institute of Psychiatry, King's College London, UK;
Honorary Consultant Psychiatrist
South London and Maudsley NHS Foundation Trust
London, UK

Sir Simon Wessely

Professor of Psychological Medicine
Institute of Psychiatry, King's College London, UK;
Honorary Consultant Psychiatrist
South London and Maudsley NHS Foundation Trust
London, UK

and

Sir Robin Murray

Professor of Psychiatric Research
Institute of Psychiatry, King's College London, UK;
Honorary Consultant Psychiatrist
South London and Maudsley NHS Foundation Trust
London, UK

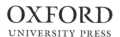

OXFORD
UNIVERSITY PRESS

OXFORD
UNIVERSITY PRESS

Great Clarendon Street, Oxford, OX2 6DP,
United Kingdom

Oxford University Press is a department of the University of Oxford.
It furthers the University's objective of excellence in research, scholarship,
and education by publishing worldwide. Oxford is a registered trade mark of
Oxford University Press in the UK and in certain other countries

Fourth edition published in 2002
Fifth edition published in 2006
Sixth edition published in 2014

Published in the United States of America by Oxford University Press
198 Madison Avenue, New York, NY 10016, United States of America

British Library Cataloguing in Publication Data
Data available

Library of Congress Control Number: 2014932183

ISBN 978–0–19–966170–1

Printed in Great Britain by
Ashford Colour Press Ltd, Gosport, Hampshire

Preface to the sixth edition

For this edition, two of the three editors, Professor Sir Simon Wessely and Dr Gareth Owen, are new, and they have been largely responsible for reviewing the entire text and bringing it up to date throughout. Once more, we have drawn upon the clinical experience of colleagues associated with the Maudsley Hospital. For this edition, we want to give special thanks to Drs John Moriarty, Larry Rifkin, Sarah Bernard, Marco Picchioni, Marta Di Forti, Jacqueline Phillips Owen, and Alex Thomson. We also want to thank Drs Sean Cross, Mike Kelleher, Ricardo Sainz Fuertes, Livia Martucci, Lisa Conlan, and Asanga Fernando. Thomas Hindmarch read the proofs on his medical elective and gave useful advice on language for upcoming doctors.

Although this book is primarily aimed at psychiatrists in training, we hope it will be useful to any clinician interested in psychiatry.

We have preserved the form of the Handbook and many of the changes to the content are fairly minor. The book is now reduced to ten chapters with revisions and updates mainly to chapters on the psychosocial assessment of adults, neuropsychiatric assessment, special problems, and treatment. Much has changed in mental health law since the last edition and we have produced a new chapter on this.

As before, responsibility for the final text rests entirely with ourselves as editors.

Gareth Owen
Simon Wessely
Robin Murray

Contents

Detailed contents

List of abbreviations

A&E	Accident and Emergency
ACE	Addenbrooke's Cognitive Examination
AMHP	approved mental health professional
AMT	Abbreviated Mental Test
ASW	approved social worker
AUDIT	Alcohol Use Disorders Identification Test
BMI	body mass index
BNF	British National Formulary
BP	blood pressure
CAMHS	Child and Adolescent Mental Health Service
CATIE	Clinical Antipsychotic Trials for Intervention Effectiveness
CBT	cognitive–behavioural therapy
CFI	Cultural Formulation Interview
CJD	Creutzfeldt–Jakob disease
CNS	central nervous system
CPA	Care Programme Approach
CPN	community psychiatric nurse
CSA	childhood sexual abuse
CSF	cerebrospinal fluid
CT	computed tomography
CTO	Community Treatment Order
CUtLASS	Cost Utility of the Latest Antipsychotic Drugs in Schizophrenia Study
CVA	cerebrovascular accident
CXR	chest X-ray
DMC	decision-making capacity
DoLS	Deprivation of Liberty Safeguards
DSH	deliberate self-harm
DSM-5	Diagnostic and Statistical Manual of Mental Disorders (5th edition)
DTs	delirium tremens
ECG	electrocardiogram
ECT	electroconvulsive therapy
EEG	electroencephalography
EPSE	extrapyramidal side-effects

ESR	erythrocyte sedimentation rate
FBC	full blood count
FGA	first-generation antipsychotic
GBL	gamma-butyrolactone
GHB	gamma-hydroxybutyrone
GI	gastrointestinal
GP	general practitioner
HIV	human immunodeficiency virus
ICD-10	International Classification of Diseases (10th revision)
IM	intramuscular
IPT	interpersonal therapy
IQ	intelligence quotient
IV	intravenous
LFT	liver function test
LPA	lasting power of attorney
LSD	lysergic acid diethylamide
MAOI	monoamine oxidase inhibitor
MCA	Mental Capacity Act
MDMA	methylenedioxymethamphetamine
ME	myalgic encephalomyelitis
MHA	Mental Health Act
MH(R)T	Mental Health (Review) Tribunal
MMSE	Mini-Mental State Examination
MND	motor neuron disease
MRI	magnetic resonance imaging
MS	multiple sclerosis
NHS	National Health Service (UK)
NICE	National Institute for Health and Care Excellence
NMS	neuroleptic malignant syndrome
nocte	at night
NSAID	non-steroidal anti-inflammatory drugs
OCP	obsessive–compulsive phenomena
od	once a day
OST	opioid substitution therapy
PD	Parkinson's disease
po	by mouth
PR	per rectum
prn	as required
PTA	post-traumatic amnesia
PTSD	post-traumatic stress disorder

qds	four times a day
QT	distance between start of Q wave and end of T wave on ECG
RC	responsible clinician
RCT	randomized controlled trial
RLAI	risperidone long-acting injection
RMO	responsible medical officer
sc	subcutaneous
SGA	second-generation antipsychotic
SLE	systemic lupus erythematosus
SSRI	selective serotonin reuptake inhibitor
STD	sexually transmitted disease
TCA	tricyclic antidepressant
TDS	three times a day
TFT	thyroid function test
U&E	urea and electrolytes
U wave	a wave on the ECG that follows the T wave
WHO	World Health Organization

The psychiatric interview with adults

The comprehensive psychiatric interview

The psychiatric interview has many features in common with the medical interview. The main goals are to elicit the necessary information to make sense of the presenting problems, to determine whether you are able to make a diagnosis, and to try and understand the origins of the presenting problems in a particular individual (the 'formulation').

Like the rest of medicine, most of the information required for a diagnosis comes from the history rather than the examination or any investigations. However, there is another feature of the psychiatric assessment which, although important in other specialities, is more explicit in psychiatry, i.e. using the interview in obtaining a trusting relationship with the patient. Rapport can determine the information obtained at interview, set the stage for a future relationship with the patient, and is likely to effect engagement and compliance with any future treatment. This is particularly important when the patient may not feel that s/he has a problem either because of a psychotic illness or where s/he has considerable ambivalence about their desire for help such as with an eating disorder or substance abuse.

Lastly, the psychiatric interview can have value both as a psychotherapeutic and psychoeducational intervention.

Recording information elicited from the interview

Modern psychiatric practice means that patients are seen in a wide variety of settings. In addition, technological change in health systems has meant that in many places electronic notes have replaced the written record. This is a trend that is likely to accelerate and expand. It is therefore no longer always possible to keep written records of the patient interview. However, the general principle remains that a record should be made as soon as possible, and as accurately as possible.

Preparing for the interview

Prior to the interview, one should review any previous records that are available. The consultation usually follows a referral from another health professional or agency. Often, a patient is already known to mental health services and may have an extensive history. It is important to review the information available so that questions are not unnecessarily repeated and essential information is not missed. It is frustrating to a patient to be repeatedly asked the same questions when that information is already in their notes.

The interview

After introducing yourself and asking the patient how they wish to be addressed, give an indication of about how long the interview may take. If relatives are present, check with the patient if they wish the relatives to attend the interview or are agreeable to them joining the interview at some point, either at the beginning or later. Patients will have a range of preferences, and judgements about the interview will need to be made on an individual basis depending on circumstances, the setting, the nature of the presenting problems, and the patient's capacity. Generally, it is best to see adult patients alone for at least a period of the interview.

Explain to the patient that if at any time they are finding the questions upsetting or would rather not answer, they should let you know. Explain that you may need to write some notes, but convey doctor–patient confidentiality. Generally, it is advisable to avoid lengthy interviews and best to collect complex information across interviews.

If the interview is for the purpose of writing a report for a third party, e.g. a court, it should be clearly stated that what is said in the interview will be put in a report and thus seen by that third party. Written consent for this should be sought unless the doctor is legally obliged to provide a report.

History of presenting complaint

The main reasons for taking a history and performing the mental state examination can be lost when starting out in psychiatry, not least because the chaos experienced by many patients is reflected in their presentation and in the telling of their story. Remember that you are taking the history and mental state so that you can make an assessment to help you plan management. This assessment goes further than making an accurate ICD-10 diagnosis, although this is crucial. Essentially, you want to answer the question 'Why has this patient presented in this way at this point in time?' Answering this will help you to form a management plan that fits your patient's needs.

Start your interview with an open question such as 'Can you tell me about the difficulties you have been having?' or 'Are there any concerns that people you know have about you?'. Try not to write anything down yet; better to be looking at the patient and listening to him/her. Only start to write after you have heard the patient's current problems and have established the order in which the various complaints developed. When you do write information down, it is essential to remember to maintain intermittent eye contact and engagement.

In taking a history, you are seeking to obtain an account of the time course and evolution of the patient's problems. This should include the social milieu within which s/he developed the problems and precipitating events. The patient's symptoms and attributions (what the patient thinks caused the symptoms) should be described, as well as how s/he tried to cope with his/her experience. The effects of any treatment taken should be noted. The effect of the patient's symptoms on his/her social functioning, occupational functioning, interpersonal functioning (family, marriage, sexual functioning, responsibility), and self-care (including eating, sleeping, weight, excretory functions, and substance use) should be described.

It is important to remember that flexibility can be required to obtain information. If a patient is very fearful, suspicious, agitated, distressed, etc., it may well be necessary to focus initially on establishing rapport by discussing their concerns or talking about non-threatening general aspects of their life. One can always return later to the main concerns that prompted the presentation once the person is more relaxed and at ease.

Precipitants
Precipitants may not emerge in the patient's spontaneous account of their problems and it is worthwhile screening for these, as it informs management plans. Specific questions may relate to:
- life events (or anniversaries of life events)
- alcohol or drug misuse
- non-adherence to medications if any have been prescribed.

Suicidal thoughts and actions
This topic is dealt with more fully in Chapter 8, 'Suicide and self-harm', p. 102. The questions form a natural hierarchy, which one goes along as far as necessary.
- Do you feel that you have a future?
- Do you feel that life's not worth living?
- Do you ever feel completely hopeless?
- Have you ever thought of ending your life?
- Have you made any plans to end your life?
- Have you made any arrangements for your affairs after your death?
- Have you ever made an attempt to take your own life?
  If 'No'—what stopped you? Relationships, faith, fear of doing it, etc.?
  If 'Yes'—can you tell me what happened?

It is essential to get an account of the frequency, intensity, and timing of suicidal thoughts, plans, or intent and the protective factors. This will enable you to understand the relation of the suicidality to the mental disorder, the times when that individual is most at risk, and to track the evolution of the suicidality over time.

For other special topics, such as alcohol and drug problems, eating disorders, epilepsy, and sexual disorder, also see Chapter 8. For organic patients, see Chapter 5.

Life charts
It is often helpful to relate events in the patient's life to illnesses that s/he has had. Life charts are especially valuable if the patient has both a physical illness and psychological problem; the columns should then be age, life event, physical illness, and psychological illness. The 'physical illness' column may of course be omitted if there is nothing to record.

In its simplest form, there is a line for each year of the patient's life; but it may be more informative to use a non-linear timescale and to give more space to some key periods of the patient's life, and less to others.

When you have finished taking the history of the present complaint, **recapitulate this history back to the patient.** Ask 'Is that right?' and 'Is there anything else I should ask you?'. At this stage, you may wish to go on to the mental state examination (Chapter 4).

Family history

The amount of detail recorded will be influenced by the nature of the patient's illness. It is important to understand that people may well be sensitive to details of family illness and particularly mental illness. It is better to first display interest in the family before enquiring about the health of the family.

It is very helpful to draw a picture of the patient's family, using squares for males and circles for females. Those who have died are indicated by an oblique line through the circle or square, together with date of death and cause of death. A double oblique line indicates marriages ended by divorce. An example is given in Figure 1.1.

You draw this figure with the patient's assistance and in full view. You then ask: 'Did anyone in your family suffer from mental health problems?' and, if so, enter details besides their symbol. This is the most informative way of collecting information about genetic loading (see Figure 1.1). If parents have separated, indicate on the family tree the age of the patient at the time when the separation occurred. Also ask about alcohol and suicide history in family members.

Personal history

This should not be a mechanical procedure, but an opportunity to understand how a character has developed. Test ideas about the patient's life, depending upon the nature of his/her current problems. Test hypotheses about the patient, using a 'negotiating' style: 'I wonder whether...'

Family background

Ask the patient to describe his/her parents or step-parents. What were they like? How did the patient get on with each of them? Where does the patient come in the sibship, and what are the achievements of each sib?

Family atmosphere

Ask about the general experience of being a child in that family. Were they happy times? If not, what was the problem? Ask about early childhood difficulties and general development. (See also Chapter 3.)

Infancy and childhood

Were there birth difficulties? Was the patient separated from his/her mother in early life? (From informant: was mother depressed after birth?)

Who brought the patient up and where? What was the occupation of the parents or care-giver? What was the general nature and quality of the relationship with each? Did the patient have any adverse or abusive experiences—physical punishment, neglect, sexual abuse?

School

Did the patient have many friends? How popular? What was his/her age on leaving school and qualifications? How did the patient get on with teachers? Was s/he encouraged by teachers? How self-confident was s/he at school? Was the patient bullied? Did s/he play truant?

Occupational history

This provides an opportunity to judge whether the patient realized his/her potential, and whether s/he has persistence. Frequent changes of job or leaving many jobs without good reason suggest an abnormal personality.

Age at first job? General areas of employment? Periods of unemployment and why? Frequency of job change? Current job—enjoyable, any problems?

Psychosexual history

Current 'partner', time with that person, difficulties, are they supportive? Previous partners. Any unwanted sexual experiences? Any unsafe sex? If the patient has a steady partner, ask about the relationship. Any children (details)?

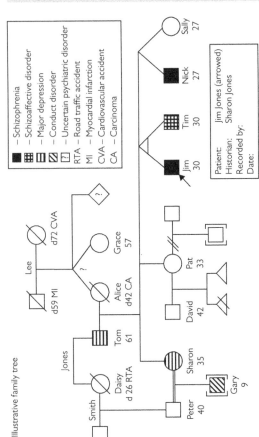

Illustrative family tree

■ – Schizophrenia
⊞ – Schizoaffective disorder
▥ – Major depression
▨ – Conduct disorder
◨ – Uncertain psychiatric disorder
RTA – Road traffic accident
MI – Myocardial infarction
CVA – Cardiovascular accident
CA – Carcinoma

Patient: Jim Jones (arrowed)
Historian: Sharon Jones
Recorded by:
Date:

Fig. 1.1 Illustrative family tree.

List of symbols used in family trees

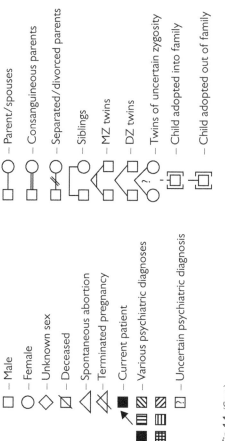

- Male
- Female
- Unknown sex
- Deceased
- Spontaneous abortion
- Terminated pregnancy
- Current patient
- Various psychiatric diagnoses
- Uncertain psychiatric diagnosis

- Parent/spouses
- Consanguineous parents
- Separated/divorced parents
- Siblings
- MZ twins
- DZ twins
- Twins of uncertain zygosity
- Child adopted into family
- Child adopted out of family

Fig. 1.1 (Cont.)

Past psychiatric history
Illnesses, hospital admissions, treatments, and episodes of self-harm.

Past and current medical and surgical history
Co-morbid physical illness is common in older patients and must be comprehensively assessed. All current medication, both regular and 'as required', should be documented. A collateral history from the patient's general practitioner (GP) may be helpful. The patient's view of his/her own health may be an important feature in the presenting complaint.

Alcohol use
All patients should be asked about their alcohol consumption. Screening aims to detect whether an alcohol problem is present and, if so, whether it is likely to respond to brief intervention or to require specialized treatment. Some commonly used screening questions are derived from the Alcohol Use Disorders Identification Test (AUDIT) (see Appendix 1).

- How often do you have a drink containing alcohol?
- How many drinks containing alcohol do you have on a typical day when you are drinking?
- How often do you have six or more drinks on one occasion?

These questions can be made less threatening by being incorporated into an assessment of general health/lifestyle or into the medical history.

Drug misuse
All patients should be asked about their use of illicit or over-the-counter drugs. However, for most patients a few brief screening questions will suffice.

- Are there any other tablets or medicines that you take, apart from those you get from your doctor?
- Is there anything you buy from the chemist or get from friends or over the internet?
- Have you used any (illegal and legal but psychoactive) drugs such as cannabis, khat, amphetamines/speed, ecstasy, cocaine/crack, LSD/acid, or heroin?
- What about tablets to settle your nerves or to help you sleep (such as temazepam or diazepam) or to enhance your performance (such as methylphenidate)?

Medication
Ask about current medication. Any allergies or problems with medication?

Forensic history
Ever had trouble with the police, trouble with the law? Date, type of offence as charged, court appearance, verdict, and sentence (custodial, probation, etc.). Attitude to offending and punishment; experience in prison.

Social history
Accommodation, finances, home activities, outside activities, carers (for fuller details, see Chapter 2, 'Assessing the social state', p. 27).

Premorbid personality
Before you became unwell what were you like? Prompt patient for whether s/he had many friends. Could s/he trust people? What was his/her temper like? How did s/he cope with life? How did s/he deal with criticism? Was s/he very tidy? (Remember that information from informants about personality is essential to build a more accurate picture.)

The comprehensive psychiatric interview has traditionally formed the part 1 summary of a hospital assessment or an assessment in a specialist clinic. Whilst every psychiatrist should be able to conduct a comprehensive psychiatric interview, and return to it as needed, interviews will often be more problem oriented and contextualized. The techniques of assessment and management described in this book are equally applicable outside the hospital (e.g. in the patient's home, a hostel or day centre, a police station, or even the street). However, some special considerations apply.

The A&E setting

Obtaining background information will enhance the efficiency and effectiveness of the assessment as well as promoting greater safety, but lays the clinician open to bias. In many situations, information can be extensive, in the form of past records (particularly electronic records) and information from the person(s) accompanying the individual. Background information becomes particularly important in the context of the psychiatric emergency.

The most common psychiatric examination the trainee will have to undertake is the emergency assessment in A&E. Commonly, a nurse will have taken the referral and there will be some triage before the doctor is contacted.

Obtain as much information as possible. This can be grouped into:
- patient identification, e.g. name, date of birth
- physical health problems (past and current, including medication)
- mental health problems (past, current assessment, and medication)
- risk to self and risk to others (past and current)
- contact details of the referrer in case you need to speak with them again; agree with the referrer where and when the patient will be seen.

Preparation of the room

Ideally, the room should be quiet, well lit, private, and with a writing surface. Safety issues must always routinely be considered before seeing every patient; these include the following (see also Chapter 7).
- Never sit the patient so that you are hemming him/her in. The furniture should be arranged such that it is easy for either of you to leave.
- Remove from sight any object that might be used as a weapon
- If there is a panic button in the room, know where it is, how it works, and whether or not it will summon aid after hours. If there is no panic button, know how to summon help.
- Avoid using rooms that are in an isolated area.
- Inform nursing colleagues what you are doing and how long you expect to be.
- If you believe that there is a more than usual risk, arrange for several (nursing) colleagues to be close at hand. Before the interview, discuss your concerns and how to manage an unwanted event.

A history of the present symptoms and a focused mental state examination are essential, as well as detailed enquiry about drugs and medications taken (or not taken) recently. Previous psychiatric history should be covered briefly, and effort should be made to collect information from others who may be accompanying the patient or available on the telephone.

The doctor will wish to admit all those whose illness represents a threat either to themselves or to others, unless satisfactory alternative care arrangements are available. Re-admissions of psychotic patients can sometimes be prevented if the keyworker is available, or if resources permit, a very brief stay in a community hostel while medication is resumed may be preferred.

Outpatient settings

This can be in community mental health teams, outpatient departments of hospitals, or GP practices. Sharing and discussing a formulation and management plan in more detail is important. It may be necessary to complete your information gathering from other sources before entering this stage. If a relative is available, ask the patient whether s/he minds if you see them. (A parent of a child under 16 has a legal right to see you, but patients over the age of 16 can object.) Use your judgement about whether to have the relative in the room while the management plan is communicated to the patient. Other things being equal, it is usually to be preferred, as the relative's attitude to what you propose is likely to be a critical factor in determining adherence, and the patient may not remember everything that you say.

Ask the patient how s/he expected that you would help them. If his/her expectations sound reasonable, give him/her details of what you think would be the best course and ask him/her whether that sounds reasonable.

If the patient's expectations are quite different from your own, explain your reasons for preferring a different course of action. A relative, if present, is often very useful at this point. Give your advice in small quantities, and get the patient to agree with what you are saying.

If the patient needs an **investigation**, explain why, what it will involve, and what steps s/he needs to take to get it done. If you are referring the patient to a colleague, tell him/her your colleague's name and the reason for the referral.

If you are **prescribing a medication** discuss:
- the main effects of the medication
- its side effects
- how long they are likely to have to take it
- whether there is a discontinuation syndrome
- whether it is habit-forming.

If you are suggesting a **course of therapeutic interviews** (or a referral for psychotherapy), discuss with the patient:
- how many interviews
- how long each will last
- what the purpose of the interviews will be
- what you expect the patient to discuss during them.

Home visits

Visiting people at home provides an invaluable insight into the social context of the patient's psychopathology and his/her level of functioning and is now routine in the UK for 'home treatment teams'.

Patients may also be seen at home as part of a traditional 'domiciliary visit' request by the GP, planned community treatment or review, as an emergency intervention in a crisis, or in a formal MHA assessment. Family assessment and intervention may very usefully be carried out in the home. CPA reviews may be held in non-medical settings. Generally, home visiting should be part of the work of the multidisciplinary mental health team.

Planning the visit

The reasons for and expected outcome of any community visit should be identified. If hospital admission is the expected outcome of an emergency assessment, the availability of a bed should be confirmed before setting out. Alternatively, the possibilities of intensive community support to an acutely ill patient should be explored prior to the visit. If the patient is likely to require medication, is a prescription available? A mobile telephone can be used to make arrangements and to contact the patient if you get lost or delayed or have difficulty in gaining access. The phone can also be used to get collateral information. The visiting psychiatrist should have the maximum possible information. It is helpful to know the exact nature of the community concerns before any doorstep assessment:

- What is the alleged psychopathology?
- What abnormal behaviours have others reported?
- What are the patient's documented risks to self or others?

The safety of any home visit should always be considered before undertaking it. The patient's notes, including recent mental state, behaviour, and risk should be read. Do not visit alone for cases that are high risk. High-risk visits include visits to, for example:

- unknown people threatening violence
- known people with a past history of serious violence, now refusing to engage with services
- known people with no history of violence, but now unwell and threatening violence
- people who it has been reported are actively attempting suicide and require an urgent home visit
- people known to be intoxicated with drugs or alcohol and at high risk of self-harm
- people who live with others with a history of violence or drug or alcohol abuse.

In such cases, consider whether the patient can visit the team base where the environment is more predictable and help is on hand or consider what other professionals need to be present at the home visit to keep it safe (e.g. the police and/or ambulance).

Carrying out a visit

Communications should be clear and unambiguous. Certain courtesies should be observed; for example, seeking permission to enter the house

and establishing with the patient and any carer the purpose of the interview, its likely duration, and where it should be carried out. Introductions
should be made. The composition of the household should be established;
visitors should be sensitive to the needs of children in the home. When
carers are present, they should be allowed to contribute to the discussion
of the patient's problems, although rights to confidentiality should always
be considered. It may be appropriate to interview the patient and carers
separately. It is quite reasonable to ask the patient to turn off the television
or remove his/her pet from the interview setting. If one aim of the visit is to
assess the patient's level of functioning and home environment, this should
be carried out sensitively, although it is usually appropriate to share any
concerns about welfare with the patient.

At the end of the visit, a plan of further care should be negotiated with
the patient and carer. Preferably, the timing of any further home visit or outpatient contact should be agreed. Details of a contact person, address, and
telephone number should be offered to the patient and carer. The referrer
should be contacted following an assessment, which should be recorded in
the case notes. It will often be helpful to carry out a short discussion with
any accompanying colleague immediately after the visit, both to clarify the
outcome of the visit and for emotional support.

Assessment of the elderly patient

This is essentially the same as that of younger adults, but there are differences of emphasis that need consideration. Assessment is frequently complicated by **cognitive impairment, physical ill-health, and frailty**, including
hearing and visual disability. As a consequence, it may be necessary to carry
out the assessment over several sessions and essential to obtain a **collateral
history** from a close relative or carer. The initial assessment will usually be
carried out in the patient's own home.

Psychiatric illness in the elderly is much like that in younger adults and
includes neurosis, personality disorders, and substance misuse. However, it
is more concerned with four major diagnoses: dementia, delirium, depression, and delusional disorder.

History of the presenting complaint

Bear in mind that some patients with dementia or delirium may lack awareness of illness. Direct questioning about memory function may be a helpful
way of beginning.

- Do you have any difficulty with your memory?
- Do you forget where you have left things more than you used to?
- Do you think that your memory is worse than that of other people of
  your age?

Other cognitive problems, such as dysphasia, dyspraxia, and agnosia, should
also be asked about (see Chapter 5, 'Mental state examination', p. 69).

Elderly patients may not admit to feeling 'depressed' or 'low in spirits'.
Careful questioning about other depressive symptoms, such as suicidal
ideas, diurnal variation, low self-esteem, hopelessness, guilt, insomnia, anorexia, and weight loss, will assist with making the diagnosis.

Paranoid or psychotic features may need to be elicited directly.

- Do you get on well with your neighbours or have you had any difficulty with them?
- Do you ever hear/see things that other people do not?
- Are people spying on you or plotting against you?
- Are people stealing from you?

Many patients with dementia present to psychiatric services because of associated psychotic, affective, or behavioural disturbances, rather than the cognitive problems. **These are best elicited from an informant.** Common psychotic symptoms in dementia include:

- delusions of theft, persecution
- auditory and visual hallucinations
- misidentification syndromes.

Common behavioural problems include:

- wandering
- aggression
- urinary incontinence
- disinhibition.

Ask whether symptoms had a sudden or gradual onset. The order in which symptoms developed is sometimes important, for example in differentiating depression with cognitive impairment from 'real' dementia or in differentiating between different types of dementia.

Cognitive assessment

Where the patient permits formal testing, a short cognitive screening test such as the Abbreviated Mental Test (AMT) or the Mini-Mental State Examination (MMSE) can be used. The Addenbrooke's Cognitive Examination (ACE) (Appendix 2) gives a more complete cognitive assessment that includes the MMSE. For patients known to have dementia, the MMSE is helpful in giving an approximate idea of the severity of impairment. A high score may provide evidence against substantial cognitive impairment. It may also be helpful in future assessments to have an idea of previous function (and therefore it is important that, where possible, previous assessments are accessed, to put any current score in context). It is vital to take previous education, levels of literacy, and sensory deficits into account when interpreting scores from these screening tests. For example, someone with high educational attainment may have clinically evident dementia and still achieve a maximum score on the MMSE. In addition, both screening tests have poor cross-cultural validity, and results should be interpreted with appropriate caution.

Cognitive screening tests such as the MMSE provide relatively little information concerning specific cognitive deficits. For example, memory impairment cannot be adequately assessed through the recall of three words. Frontal lobe function is also poorly assessed by this instrument. Both memory and frontal lobe function are better assessed with the ACE. If cognitive impairment is suspected, a formal assessment should be carried out as outlined in Chapter 4.

Family history

Enquire about the family as a source of support. Ask about a history in first-degree relatives of:
- dementia, Parkinson's disease, mental illness
- heart or stroke disease, hypertension
- cancer
- Down's syndrome.

Personal history

Sexual activity should be asked about in a straightforward and direct way. It should not be assumed that sexual behaviour will have ceased simply because a person is old.

Ask about reaction to life events:
- retirement
- bereavement
- serious illness in the patient or a close relative.

Elder abuse is increasingly recognized. The following neutral series of questions may allow further exploration of this difficult area:
- Has anyone shouted at or insulted you recently?
- Has anyone hit you or handled you roughly recently?
- Has anyone stopped you getting the help you need recently?

Social history

This follows the usual schema outlined in Chapter 2, 'Assessing the social state', p. 27. However, important areas in the elderly, other than housing and finance, include the following:
- Social network: what support is there from family/friends, clubs? What day centres are attended and how frequently?
- Home-care support: does the patient receive meals-on-wheels, home helps, and district nurses? How frequently? Are they helpful?

Lastly, an account of the patient's ability to perform activities of daily living should be obtained. This should include information on the following:
- Mobility: the use of walking aids; whether stairs can be climbed without help.
- Personal hygiene: washing, continence, using the toilet, and dressing. For example: can you wash yourself without help? Do you have trouble controlling your bladder? Can you dress yourself without help?
- Domestic activities: cooking, laundry, housework, and paying bills.

Taking a collateral history

Attempts should be made to obtain a collateral history for all psychiatric assessments. In the case of older patients, the following information may be most accurately obtained from an informant:
- history of cognitive decline
- onset, e.g. forgetfulness, and course of cognitive decline, if suspected
- personality change (suggestive of frontal lobe pathology)
- behavioural disturbance associated with cognitive decline
- activities of daily living and level of support.

In the presence of confabulation, ascertaining deficits in long-term memory, as part of the mental state examination, may be impossible without an informant.

In the collateral history, it is particularly important to investigate the extent of carer strain. This may be a component in the patient's presentation, is an important risk factor for elder abuse, and may affect later treatment decisions and prognosis.

Home visits to elderly patients

If the patient is being assessed at home, some inspection of the home circumstances should be made. This is an important part of evaluating the degree of risk posed to the patient (and possibly others). Remember that self-neglect is not diagnostic of any particular disorder and can occur in severe functional illness as well as dementia.

* Is the dwelling in a good state of repair and decoration?
* Is it secure?
* Are gas, electricity, and water connected?
* Is there adequate heating and lighting?
* Is the gas ever left on unlit?
* If the patient smokes, is there evidence of the careless use of lit cigarettes?
* Is the patient able to call for help if necessary (e.g. via a centralized alarm system)?
* Is there enough food in the home to make, at least, small snacks/hot drinks?
* Is there evidence of urinary or faecal incontinence?
* Are any pets well cared for?

Psychosocial assessments with adults

Assessing early life experience

Suitable informants may be necessary for assessing early life experience. The patient may only be able to report what they have been told about their early years, the period of normal childhood amnesia. If they report amnesia for most of their childhood, there must be a strong suspicion that there have been events too painful to remember which have been either repressed or, alternatively, the patient is not at this moment willing to relate. Significant events that probably will have influenced a person's early development, coping strategies, personality, relationship patterns, and vulnerabilities are as follows:

1. Puerperal illness of the mother, leading to actual separation or subtle deficiencies in early maternal care.
2. Death of a parent and bereavement reactions of the survivors can have a lasting effect. Who helped the child to mourn?
3. Chronic illness, especially mental illness of a parent. Was it a family secret? What help did the family have from outside? Did the child have to take a parental role?
4. Parental strife and separation leading to divided loyalties. A mother who cannot separate from a violent partner exposes her children to confusion. They want to but cannot protect her, and they cannot understand why she does not leave to protect herself.
5. Single parenthood: poverty, lack of emotional support, frequent changes of sexual partner, increased risk of child abuse by partners.
6. Frequent changes of domicile: ruptures peer relationships and disrupts schooling.
7. Bullying at school suggests poor self-esteem, poor social skills, and insecure early attachment pattern.
8. Frequent hospitalizations: separations, painful operations, disruption of schooling and peer relations, over-protective or emotionally detached parents.
9. Major environmental failure: in and out of care, foster homes, children's homes, childhood sexual and physical abuse, neglect, emotional deprivation.

Memories of sexual abuse

There is now compelling evidence from well-conducted case-control studies that childhood sexual abuse (CSA) is followed by higher rates of depression and anxiety during childhood and early adult life, greater incidence of deliberate self-harm, and eating disorders during adolescence and early adult life. Since sexual abuse of children is commonly accompanied by both physical abuse and poor care—and can be followed by numerous adverse events—it is difficult to disentangle the specific psychiatric effects of each kind of abuse. Drug and alcohol abuse are important long-term sequelae of CSA as is continuing low self-esteem. A dose effect appears to operate, relating severity of CSA to severity of adult psychopathology, and CSA is a risk factor for adults with post-traumatic stress disorder (PTSD), dissociation, and psychotic symptoms.

Not all patients who give vivid descriptions of sexual abuse have in fact been abused, and false memories are especially likely to occur after misguided 'therapeutic' efforts to recover such memories. The situation is complicated by the fact that some people who were actually abused have repressed their memories of the abuse, a fact that leads some self-styled therapists to embark on sometimes ill-advised treatment designed to recover such memories. It is also important to recognize the surprisingly high population rates of contact abuse in under 18s with estimates between 27–38 per cent in females and around 11 per cent of males.

Psychiatric practice and memories of sexual abuse

Obtaining a psychiatric history which may include sexual abuse poses difficulties. Repeated admissions to psychiatric hospitals leads to the history being recounted on many occasions. What we know about memory is that if there is extensive rehearsal of an imagined event, the person can believe the event happened. The memory can become highly detailed and vivid to the person. The event can be altered in matters of detail by suggestion and leading questions. It is common practice for the patient's account to be recorded in psychiatric notes without any attempt to question the source or reliability of the memory. Indeed, an American Psychiatric Association report (2000) stated:

> Psychiatrists should maintain *an empathic, non-judgmental, neutral stance* towards memories of sexual abuse. As in the treatment of all patients, care must be taken to avoid prejudging the cause of the patient's difficulties or the veracity of the patient's reports. A strong belief by the psychiatrist that sexual abuse, or other factors, are or are not the cause of the patient's problems is likely to interfere with appropriate assessment and treatment. Many individuals who have experienced sexual abuse have a history of not being believed by their parents, or others in whom they have put their trust. Expression of disbelief is likely to cause the patient further pain and decrease his/her willingness to seek psychiatric treatment. Similarly clinicians should not exert pressure on patients to believe in events that may have not occurred, or to prematurely disrupt important relationships or make other important decisions based on these speculations.

One of the strongest criteria in assessing the reliability of a memory is the accuracy with which it is anchored in place and time. However, it may be difficult to establish these sorts of facts in the context of the approach (empathic non-judgemental) defined by the American Psychiatric Association. Thus, the history from the patient may be unreliable and the process of repeated psychiatric history taking may further contribute to faulty recollection.

Absent memories: amnesia for abuse

In one study, children who had presented for medical care immediately following sexual abuse were seen as adults on average 17 years later. Over a third (38 per cent) appeared to have no memory of their early abuse.

Loss of memory was most common if the abuse occurred when they were young and was perpetrated by someone they knew.

Normal memory

To a degree, all memories are unreliable. They are not held like video tapes in the mind to be replayed at recall. Rather, when a memory is cued it is processed even prior to the stage it reaches awareness. This processing can include the incorporation of general knowledge or material from another record. Following the remembering, information will be stored as a record of the remembering. The next time the cycle of remembering is entered, the recall may be for the original, or may be for the previous recall. Not every detail of an event is stored in memory. When an event is recalled it might need elaborating before it is intelligible to consciousness. What we are conscious of is a mixture of reproduction and reconstruction. Reconstructive memory is characterized by conflation of different events, filling out detail, and importation of information. Nothing can be recalled accurately from before the first birthday and little from before the second. Poor memory from before the fourth birthday is normal.

The factors which influence the degree of reconstruction include:
- the personal significance of the event
- its emotive content
- the time elapsed between the event occurring and its recall
- the age at which the event occurred
- the reasons why the person is remembering the event and the circumstances of recall.

False beliefs and incorrect memories

There is a great deal of evidence for incorrect memories in 'normal' mental states, i.e. where an event has happened but the details are wrongly recalled and there is an unstable relationship between confidence and accuracy.

Abnormal mental states are likely to lead to other kinds of errors in the reconstruction of memories. This is obvious in psychotic states but also occurs in extreme emotional states.

In the context of CSA, normal human tendencies toward false beliefs and incorrect memories need to be balanced against the evidence that people who have been abused are often not believed when they speak of it. Experts tend to agree that children who spontaneously describe CSA and make an intentional disclosure are likely to be accurate but also that suggestive interviewing can create marked inaccuracies.

Informants

The fact that memories can be unreliable is recognized in psychiatry and is why informants are often used to corroborate the history. This is acknowledged as good psychiatric practice. The history should be compiled from information elicited both from the patient and from one or more informants. The informant's account will not only amplify the patient's report of factual detail but will supplement the patient's account. The corroborative evidence that is useful in a psychiatric history is different from that required for forensic reasons. Open, broad questions can be used. For example, if there is a history of CSA, it would be reasonable to ask the parents, other relatives, and schools whether any difficulties or concerns were noted during the child's development. CSA is recognized as 'significant harm' in the Children Act (1989). Legal duties relating to safeguarding children are outlined in Chapter 10, 'Children Act 1989', p. 170.

Reference

American Psychiatric Association (2000). Therapies focused on memories of childhood physical and sexual abuse. *American Journal of Psychiatry*, **157**(10), 1722.

Assessing personality

Why assess personality?

Premorbid personality colours the presentation of mental illness. In addition, personality is one of the determinants of illness behaviour and adherence to treatment. Therefore, the assessment of premorbid personality is an essential part of a psychiatric assessment. Furthermore, personality disorders are common and burdensome conditions. Epidemiological research has shown that the prevalence of personality disorders steadily increases with each level of care: 10 per cent in the community, 20 per cent in primary care, and 30–60 per cent among samples of psychiatric patients as a main or ancillary diagnosis. People with a personality disorder have an increased risk of suicide, accidents, mental illnesses such as depression, and drug misuse, and respond less well to treatment than people without personality disorder. They are heavy users of health services and are, therefore, frequently encountered in clinical practice.

Definitions

Personality is a term used to describe enduring traits and behaviours that differentiate individuals from each other. Personality traits are usually present since adolescence, stable over time (with accentuation under stress), and evident in a range of different environments. Personality disorders, on the other hand, are mental disorders characterized by enduring patterns of inner experience and behaviour that deviate from the individual's culture and are pervasive and inflexible. A core, defining feature of personality disorders is that the traits and linked behaviour are associated with significant personal, social, or occupational impairment. The ICD-10 categories of personality correspond roughly to the DSM-5 categories. DSM recognizes three 'clusters' of personality disorder, brief details of which are given in Table 2.1.

Table 2.1 Clusters of personality disorders from DSM-5

Cluster A ('odd or eccentric' types)	Paranoid, schizoid, and schizotypal personality disorders
Cluster B ('dramatic, emotional, or erratic' types)	Histrionic, narcissistic, antisocial, and borderline personality disorders
Cluster C ('anxious and fearful' types)	Obsessive–compulsive, avoidant, and dependent

The three clusters are used widely by clinicians and have been shown to be useful in distinguishing different populations of psychiatric patients (Reich and Thompson 1987). Cluster B—the dramatic cluster—presents most often to psychiatric services. The main features are:

- Borderline: mood instability (often across minutes, hours, or a few days); impulsivity; self-harm; intense and unstable relationships with patterns of idealization/devaluation, spitting, and efforts to avoid real or imagined abandonment; unclear, diffuse identity; chronic feelings of emptiness. There is often overlap with depression, anxiety, substance abuse, and eating disorder.
- Histrionic: self-dramatization; inappropriate seductiveness; over-concern with physical appearance; suggestibility; seeking excitement and to be centre of attention; shallow and labile affectivity; manipulative behaviours.
- Narcissistic: grandiosity; fantasies of unlimited success; sense of entitlement; envious; arrogant, haughty behaviours; need for admiration.
- Antisocial: callous lack of concern for others, disregard and violation of others' rights; aggression; evidence of childhood conduct disorder.

Categories or dimensions?

Doctors tend to prefer the use of categories when describing abnormal states. However, the categorical model of personality disturbance has its limitations. Criteria for categories of personality disorder frequently overlap, and clinicians often disagree on whether categories are present or not. In fact, personality is probably more accurately conceptualized in terms of variation along the 'Big Five' dimensions of neuroticism, extroversion, openness to experience, agreeableness, and conscientiousness (Digman 1990). However, although the research evidence favours dimensions, categories lead more readily to treatment decisions and convey more vividly the disturbance demonstrated by the highly abnormal people that psychiatrists are called on to assess.

Use the term 'personality disorder' cautiously!

People with personality disorders are often the most difficult patients to be encountered in clinical practice. They often intrude directly on staff feelings. It is important to avoid using the term 'personality disorder' merely to explain disagreeable behaviour. There are stigmatizing effects of applying the label of personality disorder. Therefore, before the diagnosis is made, positive evidence must be sought. When this is done it can become possible to share the findings with the patient who is sometimes relieved to have their difficulties described accurately. Successful communication is aided by having psychological frameworks for treatment available and by taking an interest in the person rather than just the 'personality disorder'.

Who should provide information?

Self-description is difficult and, in a clinical situation, the presence of affective disorder or psychosis may distort the assessment of personality. For these reasons, in addition to the patient's account of him or herself, it is also desirable to obtain a corroborative account from an informant. The informant should be someone who has known the patient when free of symptoms for a number of years and preferably in more than one circumstance. The interview should enquire into positive as well as negative aspects of the patient's personality, as these may also guide the management strategy.

How should the interview proceed?

It is important to be sure that the informant or patient (as his or her own informant) understands that this interview concerns a time of life when the patient was well. Agree on that time (e.g. 5 years ago or before the marriage broke down) and focus the interview on that period. Begin by asking the informant an open-ended question, to describe in his or her own words how the patient was at that time. This response itself may indicate which diagnostic category of personality may be appropriate. However, if uninformative, the following more specific questions will probe for one of the ICD-10 categories.

Start your discussion of personality with a general screening question, such as 'How does she or he get on with other people?'. Go on to the questions listed in Table 2.2, asking clarifying questions only if you have a positive reply to a screening question.

Table 2.2 Screening and clarifying questions for personality disorder

Screening question (group)	Clarifying questions
Does s/he trust other people? (paranoid)	Is s/he a suspicious person who misinterprets the actions of others as threatening or demeaning?
	Does s/he consistently bear grudges?
Would you describe him/her as a loner? (schizoid)	Does s/he almost always prefer to do solitary things?
	Is s/he a detached, aloof, or cold person?
Does s/he have difficulty controlling his/her temper? (dissocial)	Is s/he consistently irresponsible?
	Does s/he lack remorse when s/he has done something wrong?
Is s/he impulsive? (emotionally unstable)	Does s/he have an unstable mood?
	Does s/he make frantic efforts to avoid abandonment?
Does s/he dislike situations where s/he is not the centre of attention (histrionic)	Is s/he a dramatic or theatrical person?
	Do his/her emotions change rapidly (over the course of minutes or hours, not days)?
Is s/he a worrier or a shy person? (anxious)	Does s/he view him/herself as inferior compared with others?
	Is s/he unwilling to become involved with people unless s/he is certain of being liked?
Does s/he depend on others a lot? (dependent)	Does s/he allow others to make the most of his/her important decisions?
	Does s/he have difficulty expressing disagreement with others for fear of rejection?
Does s/he have unusually high standards at work or home? (anankastic)	Is s/he so preoccupied with details and rules that the main point of an activity is lost?
	Does s/he insist that others do things the way s/he wants them to be done?

Any one of these probes may point to one of the ICD-10 categories. Therefore, the interviewer should follow with subsidiary questions that concern the additional features of that category (see ICD-10 for further details). In addition, the informant should be asked to indicate whether these features were generally present (e.g. not just at work) and whether the personality seemed responsible for personal suffering (e.g. periods of distress or unhappiness) or handicap in social or occupational life. From this information, abnormal premorbid personality may be identified or personality disorder diagnosed. If the patient is to be the informant, then the same procedure can be followed. A number of reliable standardized assessment procedures for personality disorders now exist and, ideally, one of these should be used as part of the assessment. Examples of reliable assessment measures, developed in the UK for use in routine clinical settings, are the Standardized Assessment of Personality and the Personality Assessment Schedule.

References

Digman, J.M. (1990). Personality structure: emergence of the five-factor model. *Annual Review of Psychology*, **41**, 417–40.

Reich, J. and Thompson, W.D. (1987). DSM-III personality disorder clusters in three populations. *British Journal of Psychiatry*, **150**, 471–5.

Assessing family relationships

There are many reasons why it can be valuable to interview the family of the presenting patient (index patient), ranging from obtaining a good description of fits, fugues, and other altered states of consciousness to an examination of the family dynamics, for example to uncover possible maintaining influences in relation to the patient who relapses when a discharge date is decided. The index patient should be included in the family meeting.

As a general rule, the earlier the family can be included in the investigation and treatment of a problem the better, assuming that the patient is agreeable. It is important for the interviewer to be alert to the strengths and resources of the family who will usually have tried hard to support and help their ill member before calling in the professionals. By the time they see you, they may be feeling demoralized and helpless. They may be angry with the patient and secretly blaming themselves or each other. Under these circumstances it is crucial that you do not add to their guilt or sense of failure.

How to manage a family interview

After initial introductions and an explanation of any specialist setting (e.g. one-way screen, closed circuit television), start by thanking the family members for coming and acknowledging interruptions to school and work. Then state the purpose of the meeting by inviting them to help you to help the index patient, as indeed they are experts by virtue of having known him or her for longer and before the illness. It is usually best to start by asking for a description of the problem, being sure to hear from each member of the family how he or she sees it.

Even at this early stage one often obtains startlingly different descriptions of the problem. It is valuable to define the problem as it affects the family now, and clarify that this may be different from how the problem began. The focus at this early stage in the interview is to translate the problem (described as an attribute of the index patient) into statements about relationships and differences in relationships among the family members. At all times it is important to note their non-verbal messages: posture, eye contact, interruptions, and emotional states (detachment, fear, sadness, etc.).

One may enquire into current alliances in relation to the present problem (who feels most upset by the problem, who notices first, who becomes impatient first), obtaining a ranking of all members in relation to each question. It is very useful to track sequences of behaviour around the problem as this provides a detailed pattern of activity which is often stereotypic.

It is the family's attempt at a solution which has itself become part of the problem. By asking different family members for their explanation of how the pattern has evolved or why particular members take up particular roles in the sequence of behaviour, it is usually possible to uncover differences of opinion about what happens. It can be useful to ask what other approaches to the problem have been tried and why they were abandoned.

When you feel that you have a clear picture of how the family tries and fails to help in relation to the immediate problem, it is time to enquire into how the problem affects other aspects of the family's life together. How does the family regroup when the index patient is ill or away in hospital? Who takes over their tasks? Who misses them most? By comparing and conducting current arrangements and role assignments with those before the problem began, certain hypotheses about what function the problem serves will emerge.

The final part of an initial family interview involves establishing with the family members whether or not they are willing to continue to work together with you. You should explain that the aim is to arrive at a better understanding of the problem and finding a way either of resolving it or living with it. Alternatively, you may discover that there is such hostility towards the index patient or so much chaos, discord, or obstructiveness that it is clear that the patient will have to be helped to live apart from their family. Although painful, this is usually much better accepted by the patient if the limits of what each family member is willing to offer in terms of help and support are clear to them. For example, a couple who had both divorced and remarried had each to say to their adult chronic schizophrenic daughter, in front of one another: 'You cannot, under any circumstances, live with me.'. In this case, the uncertainty had been perpetuated by each one saying: 'Wait until you are better. Then you can live with me or possibly the other parent.'.

There is so much information to take in, record, and interpret in a family interview, that it is of great value to have a non-involved observer or a video recording. Any kind of electronic record requires the informed consent of the family at the beginning of the interview with the option to delete the recording at the end.

Your observations may be recorded under the following headings.

Description of family members present
The family includes all those living in the same household, but children who have left home and relatives in other households who are significantly involved may be included.

- Note absent members.
- List names, ages, and mental state.

Description of problem
- Use the words of family members.
- Include the problem as it began and the problem now.
- Record stereotypic pattern, if elicited.

The stage of the family life cycle
- **Courtship**, marriage, and the honeymoon period.
- The **first child** alters the couple's view of themselves and each other as they make space for the baby.
- **Subsequent children** each make demands for adjustment on existing family members.
- The **children reach adolescence** with the coming of puberty, sexual awakening, and bids for independence, and face the challenge of leaving home.
- The **empty nest**, as the last child leaves home. The couple, having reached mid-life or later, face the dependence, illness, or death of their own parents, as well as what remains of their own life together.

Crises in families often arise when transition to the next stage is required but, for some reason, cannot be successfully negotiated. Crises may result in a symptomatic member or marital difficulties, or both.

The genogram or family tree
This can be a powerful tool for eliciting transgenerational resonances. It is important to ask about stillbirths and other premature deaths; note the ages and date of death of grandparents, siblings, and children. Crises in the life cycles of the previous generation (the parents' families of origin) may illuminate difficulties in the presenting family. The occupation of each person should be indicated, if known.

The family structure
This refers to the existence of appropriate or inappropriate boundaries between different parts of the family: the boundary between the couple and each of their families of origin, as well as parents and children. Are there transgenerational alliances: father and daughter; mother and son; grandmother, mother, and daughter? Is one member of the family isolated (e.g. father) or scapegoated (e.g. a child who is different from the other siblings)? Facts informing these judgements can be elicited by asking about the routine daily activities: who does what with whom? How are mealtimes, bedtimes, housework, household chores, and leisure activities arranged? How are decisions made? Do the couple consult one another? If not, who is consulted and who is not? How are conflicts negotiated and resolved? Who has the final say? Who controls the finances? In families with an ill adolescent, the hierarchy is sometimes inverted; the parents are capriciously governed by their offspring.

Family roles and attitudes

In response to the questions above it should also become clear whether particular family members are assigned by common agreement to certain roles, and how power, authority, and gender-specific activities are distributed. Implicit in these roles will be shared attitudes, although when made explicit, differences of opinion may emerge. Acceptance of role assignment may be a way of avoiding conflict. Cultural and religious attitudes are often expressed in role assignments and expectations based on gender and birth order. A good way to find out more about cultural and religious views with which the interviewer is unfamiliar is to acknowledge difference and ignorance, and ask. It also allows the family members to describe what it is like for them to belong to an ethnic minority and the impact of the dominant culture on their lives.

Communication and emotional climate

These aspects of the description of family relationships will first of all depend upon your observations of the family as they have responded to your questioning. Supplementary questioning can clarify how the various family members experience and think about each other. For example, if the mother tends to answer for her daughter, one can ask the daughter 'Does your mother always know what you are thinking?' or ask the father or other relative 'How does your daughter manage to get her mother to speak for her?' or ask a sibling 'Does your mother always speak for your sister or are there times when your sister can speak for herself?'.

Other common patterns are as follows: one family member is frequently interrupted by another; one member is habitually silent and ignored, or disengaged, or over-emotional; everyone talks at once; no one finishes a sentence; no one listens to anyone else; one member habitually defers to another.

There may be obvious omissions or evasions. Communication may be clear and direct or contradictory and obscure.

The emotional atmosphere may be free or frozen, cool and distant, or intensely over-involved. Dyads or subsystems may be locked in superiority and submission, condescension and self-effacement, or cruelty and humiliation.

The hypothesis

Each family member is predicted to both gain and suffer from the status quo. What family member contributions maintain and prevent resolution of the problem? This is an attempt to describe the problem in systemic terms.

Assessing the social state

The social state provides a structure for supplanting and extending information that may be recorded in the history, partly under 'previous personality' and partly under 'social history' or 'current circumstances'. It comprises five main headings, for each of which four main categories of information and assessment can be reported. The four categories or columns will not all be needed if significant problems are absent. The format must allow for the possibility that only a very brief or highly distilled report will be required (or feasible) in some cases. Other reports may require a lot of detailed information.

The social state should be inserted in the notes, after the history and before the mental state examination.

Some aspects of the social state, notably culture and educational achievements, are commented on elsewhere.

Under each heading, try and distinguish between the following:

- **Facts**—aims to record the situation in terms of reported objective information from the patient or identified others (including the assessor).
- **Problems**—comprises two kinds of element, which may be reported separately: subjective difficulties reported by the patient and objective difficulties observed by others.
- **Services**—reports provisions already made at the time of assessment to alleviate some, but not necessarily all, the problems identified. Inadequacies or over-provision may be commented on, but this area of the assessment report is not the place to record proposals about management.
- **Strengths**—invites the assessor to report on positive features of the patient's social opportunities and functioning, which may serve to counterbalance the commonly prevailing negative tone of many psychiatric assessments by highlighting positive resources, relationships, and potentialities.

Accommodation

Under this heading are described the physical nature of the patient's residence and the identity of the people who normally provide the immediate social environment. The aim is to assess the type and quality of physical resources available to the patient in the home and to name the people who share the accommodation. Subheadings include the following:

- type of accommodation
- physical amenities, personal space
- quality of accommodation
- identity of other people sharing the accommodation
- ease of access
- physical security
- nature and quality of neighbourhood.

Finances

This requires a description of the patient's financial status and use of welfare benefits in order to assess income, monetary assets, liabilities, and capacities to handle money. Subheadings include the following:

- sources of income (including welfare benefits)
- capital, savings, other assets
- expenditure (including special liabilities such as gambling)
- debts (including threats of punitive action such as withdrawal of services or eviction)
- patient's contribution to, or dependence upon, the household
- budgeting capacity, including: capacity to decide financial affairs, lasting power of attorney, or court appointed deputy.

Home activities

The focus here is on daily events and activities within the home and the provision of both informal and professional support and services from people visiting the home. Subheadings include the following:

- way of spending a typical day (includes waking and rising, daily routines)
- daily living skills (including personal hygiene, laundry, cooking, cleaning)
- recreational activities.

Outside activities

The patient is seen in relationship to the local and wider community outside the home residence. Subheadings include the following:

- occupation
- social contacts (family, friends, others)
- visitors, relationships with immediate neighbours
- shopping
- travel
- use of public amenities (e.g. pubs, cinema)
- other outside leisure activities
- religious observance
- holidays.

Carer's assessment

Under this heading are listed the people who are individually identifiable as accepting a special responsibility for promoting and sustaining the patient's welfare. They may include family members, friends, other informal contacts, and members of professional agencies. Professional carers include staff members of NHS agencies (GP, psychiatric services, etc.), staff members of other statutory agencies (social services, etc.), and members of voluntary bodies (including religious organizations).

- Name, address, and telephone number of carer.
- What is the relationship with the patient?
- How long have you been the carer?
- Is the patient living with you?
- What help do you provide?
- What effect does being a carer have on you?
- Is the level of care you provide likely to change?

Cross-cultural assessments in psychiatry

The goal of the doctor–patient relationship is to achieve restoration to a state of well-being and functioning, regardless of the cultural background of the patient. However, misinterpretations of a patient's cultural beliefs concerning well-being can be an obstacle to this outcome.

In considering cultural assessment in psychiatry, we have to consider not only the race and ethnic identity of the patient (constructs lacking precise definition), but also religious and spiritual beliefs, attitudes to gender, sexual orientation, social hierarchy, lifestyle, work, etc. To assess culture is to ask the questions: 'what are the capabilities, notions and forms of behaviour this person has acquired as a *member of society*?' and 'what is the *world-view* of this person?'. Culture refers to both a basic similarity between humans (we are all cultural) and to systematic differences (our acquired habits, notions, etc. vary).

Awareness that our diagnostic systems are built from primarily specialist clinical settings using 'western' concepts and categories of human functioning, can help these systems from becoming inappropriately reified and universalized in application. Yet, awareness that psychotic behaviour, or problems resembling anxiety and depression, exists across settings that have barely heard of psychiatry (most of the world) can help prevent inappropriate assumptions that mental disorder only exists in the 'developed' or 'medicalized' world.

Cultures influence the way idioms of distress are expressed and where and when help is sought. Cultures can perpetuate symptomatology and can also influence patterns of social support. If the clinician does not know about a particular culture, it is important to find out about its essential features, including taboos, dietary restrictions, rites of passage, and religious values. However, a common pitfall is to assume that the patient's beliefs and perceptions can be solely attributed to that particular culture. This assumption neglects 'acculturation'.

Acculturation can be thought of as the adoption of customs by immigrants living in a new society. It must be seen as a multidimensional phenomenon that reflects the changes an individual goes through when she or he is exposed to a new culture—changes that can involve identity. Acculturation applies to individuals, families, religious groups, and other collectives. It is not identical at each level and it is possible that degrees of acculturation will vary across different members of the family. Acculturation can be assessed by determining the period since migration and the reasons for migration (it may be worthwhile asking about difficulties during and after migration as well as about coping and adjustment). It can also be assessed by focusing on religious activity, languages, marriage, family and gender roles, preferred dietary patterns, preferred leisure activities, aspirations, and attitudes to work and relationships.

Planning the assessment and communication

The first and preferred language in which the patient communicates must be identified as soon as practical. If this is not English, an appropriate interpreter may be required who can also act as an adviser on non-verbal communication as well as identifying idioms of distress and 'emotional' words used by the patient. Family members should not be used routinely for interpretation, and using children is fraught with particular difficulties. The selection of interpreters is central to the outcome of any assessment process and requires thought. If there is no immediate clinical need, assessment should be delayed until such time as a suitable interpreter, with objectivity and credibility, is present. If a good interpreter is found for a patient, get their name and ask to use them again for that patient.

Tact and sensitivity are important and practical gestures can make a difference. Examples include offering to remove shoes (on a home visit), not sitting with the soles of one's feet visible, not assuming a hand shake with members of the opposite sex, or offering the patient water to drink and a suitable food in hospital (e.g. access to halal, kosher, vegan). Males in some cultures will assume a hierarchical position within families or with interaction with females, and recognizing this in assessment can prevent misinterpretation.

As with assessing any patient for the first time, the initial step must be an unstructured ten minutes of 'emotional orientation', during which idioms of distress and key emotional words and terms can be identified which will give a clue towards the direction in which the assessment must proceed. Identifying the patient's term for their problem and then using it is an important way of maintaining communication, especially when the patient holds explanatory models such as spiritual or supernatural ones.

Some cultures have a great respect for the health profession, doctors in particular, such that their members may not confront, question, disagree with, or point out the problems that they may be facing. These may manifest as selective omission of medication, inaccurate reporting of symptoms, consultation with other healers who may be giving excessive reassurance or promise of a miraculous cure. Other cultures place great emphasis on native medicine and faith healers, which also may encourage patients to disengage with mental health services. It is important, wherever possible, to clarify the details of concurrent and previous faith healer/traditional healer/native medicine input, and to encourage communication between these professionals and mental health services. Often this synergy can lead to these other professionals advocating a 'mixed' approach to therapy comprising, for example, antipsychotics and prayer. Another approach that may be of value in destigmatizing mental disorder is to normalize mental disorder with physical illness. Most people, across cultures, do not think twice about undergoing an X-ray for a broken leg or taking antibiotics for a chest infection. These can be used as parallels to frame the assessment and management of mental disorder.

Cultural formulation

Semi-structured cultural assessment interviews can be useful as the basis for beginning to understand a patient's suffering in their terms and going on to develop a collaborative therapeutic relationship. Some patients, irrespective of their ethnic status, will require a longer assessment before a comprehensive formulation and management plan can be made. Some questions to help guide a cultural formulation are given in Box 2.1.

Assessing data in the history

Adverse events

Do not assume that life events, adverse or otherwise, have the same significance across cultures or that they have only the significance standardly described in the literature. Flexible enquiry will accurately elicit the impact of a patient's life events. Similarly, hospital admission or separation from children may be more adverse than one might imagine, perhaps with culturally unacceptable implications.

Psychological/somatic mindedness

In western cultures, there is often an assumption that a clear dichotomy exists between psychological and somatic symptoms, with somatization being taken to imply a lack of 'psychological mindedness'. In other cultures,

Box 2.1 Cultural formulation

Cultural definition of the problem

How would you describe your problem? How would you describe your problem to family, friends, etc.? What troubles you most about your problem? Focus on the individual's own way of understanding the problem and how they frame it for members of their social network. Use the term, expression, or brief description of the problem in subsequent questions.

Cultural perceptions of cause, context, and support

Causes: What do you think are the causes of your problem? What do others in your family, your friends, etc. think is causing your problem?

Social stresses and supports: Are there any kinds of support (e.g. from family) that make your problem better? Are there any kinds of stresses (e.g. relationships, difficulties at work) that make your problem worse?

Role of cultural identity: Are there any aspects to your background or identity that you think are making a difference to your problem? Or are causing others concern or difficulties for you?

Cultural factors affecting self-coping and past help-seeking

What have you done on your own to cope with your problem? In the past, what kind of help, advice, or healing have you sought for your problem?

Clarify the experience and regard for previous help and probe for traditional or alternative healing as required. What has got in the way to seeking help?

Cultural factors affecting current help-seeking

What kinds of help do you think would be most useful at this time for your problem? Are there kinds of help that your family, friends, etc. have suggested?

Have you been concerned with being misunderstood by doctors because of a different background? Is there anything that we can do to provide the care you need?

Adapted from the Cultural Formulation Interview (CFI) DSM-5

no such clear dichotomy is assumed. Depression in Asian, Chinese, and African cultures, for example, is expressed more somatically than in western cultures, but it would be misleading to interpret this as a lack of psychological mindedness.

Previous experience of services and treatments

Such information is helpful because previous bad experiences may deter patients from using the services optimally and engaging with them. Previous experiences may not necessarily have occurred in this country, and the criteria for help-seeking and service provisions may differ widely, thereby making the acceptability of statutory services problematic.

Racism

Members of ethnic minorities may have experienced discrimination in one or more fields of daily life, such as legal, financial, educational, or health care activities. This may be direct discrimination (wronged directly because of actions and attitudes toward one's race or ethnic group) or indirect discrimination (wronged as a result of actions, attitudes, or policies that, though not aiming at disadvantaging certain racial or ethnic groups, have the effect of disproportionately doing so). It is important to enquire about experiences of discrimination in a careful, paced, and sensitive manner so that the patient may respond accordingly. Even if perceived racist experiences do not directly contribute to the patient's presentation, these reports should be treated with respect and not dismissed as unimportant or irrelevant. If a patient finds that such experiences are not being understood or taken seriously, they may find it difficult to trust the clinician with more sensitive information.

Assessing the mental state across cultures

Assessment of the mental state must be thorough and detailed, as with any other patient. However, where the patient does not share the mental health professional's culture (regardless of skin colour), any symptoms and signs must be appraised critically in a cultural context and the appraisal revisited in response to the emergence of more information.

Behaviour

Behaviours which may appear odd or bizarre to the assessing clinician may have a culturally sanctioned role. For example, speaking in tongues, excessive religiosity, and trance possession may be culturally sanctioned. These phenomena can only be evaluated by carefully recording the behaviour, the patient's explanation for it, and the response of the family and cultural group to it. These views, if a sign of illness, may change as the patient recovers and become important signs by which the patient, their carers, and others in the folk sector may identify a relapse in the future. Unusual behaviour that is not clearly understandable should not readily be assigned as evidence of psychosis without due attention to the adaptive/coping potential of the behaviour.

Aggression

Expressions of frustration and approaches to conflict resolution show cultural variation as do cultural norms around aggression as such. The only way to assess a potentially aggressive patient, whose cultural values, norms, and mores around aggression may be different, is to first be comfortable about the safety of the assessors and of those around the patient (see Chapter 7, 'The patient who threatens violence', p. 93).

Hallucinations

The exact experiences and consistency, and especially differentiation from illusions and suggestibility states, must be ascertained. If the patient uses figures of speech inexactly to articulate their own illness experience, the clinician must avoid erroneously identifying them as hallucinations. The presence of visual phenomena are especially difficult to locate firmly within the standard psychopathology framework.

Delusions

Delusion may be a less prominent feature of descriptions of psychosis outside the west, with emphasis instead being on incoherent speech, talking to oneself, disrobing, wandering, etc. The traditional definition of delusion does take the role of culture into account. There is, of course, a possibility that if the examiner is not clear about cultural values, a delusional experience may be attributed to a culture to which it does not belong. Religious ideas, culturally sanctioned explanations, and spiritual or cosmic explanations must be carefully identified and documented verbatim. Do not just record your impressions. Always consider alternative reasons for a patient's beliefs with their relatives or advocates. Again record their responses intact. If a belief is culturally unfamiliar and is coupled with functional impairment or culturally inappropriate behaviour (relative to the patient), it is likely to be a sign of illness.

Cognitive assessment

The standard cognitive assessment may yield very little diagnostic psychopathology if used blindly across cultures, especially with different languages. It is better to obtain third-party information on the memory failure and intellectual decline. If schedules of cognitive assessment are available in the patient's primary language, these must be employed, bearing in mind the patient's level of education. Again, the help of an advocate or a team member who speaks the patient's first language can be invaluable.

Management of patients from other cultures

Cultural assessment may impact directly upon treatment. Examples range from knowing about the possibility of 'benign ethnic neutropenia' when prescribing clozapine—a possibility in people of African descent or from parts of the Middle East; to knowing what medicinal products different cultural groups use or abuse (e.g. St John's Wort in groups with beliefs in herbal remedies or Khat in people from parts of East Africa and the Middle East); to understanding the cultural appropriateness of, for example, family therapy in different parts of the world.

Overall, cultural assessment will help frame approaches to management by way of understanding the patient and their milieu, reading the signs of illness, and maintaining the doctor–patient relationship.

It is good clinical practice to discuss diagnosis and management plans with the patient and their advocates or identified family members (see Box 2.2). The appropriateness of aetiological and diagnostic concepts should be considered with an awareness of cultural norms. If the patient and other interested parties, including advocates, disagree with the intended management plan, clinicians must arrange to meet again and continue to discuss. The discussion should include mental capacity and risk assessment.

Box 2.2 Good practice points

- Be aware of your own culture and limitations.
- For each party involved in consultation, elicit first language, religion, self-defined ethnicity, identification with specific cultural groups.
- Meet with the interpreter before the assessment commences to identify their knowledge of culture, identify sources of difference (e.g. dialect, tribe, religion).
- Define and redefine terms used by you and the patient to ensure shared understanding of problems.
- Identify emotional idioms of distress and develop a shared vocabulary with the patient.
- Ask for clarification of symptoms or signs that appear unusual or unfamiliar.
- Do not be judgemental about patterns of communication or domination of the clinical interview by one family member—this may be cultural or the family style of communication.
- Be sensitive to the effects of your action, the setting, or the referral mode which jeopardize trust. Communicate confidentiality. Identify the scenario where the patient may be most comfortable and relaxed (e.g. with family versus alone).
- Be sensitive to religious and social taboos.
- Do not ask children to interpret. Avoid relatives interpreting unless it is an emergency and delay will be detrimental to the patient.
- Involve patient advocates early, with the patient's consent.
- Discuss the findings with an independent person properly familiar with the culture, within the bounds of strict confidentiality.

The psychiatric interview with children

Some differences from interviewing adults

1. The child is *brought*: the reasons may not have been explained or they may be inaccurate. The child may believe s/he is going to be told off, taken away, kept, or hurt. They may be waiting for a blood test or operation.
2. The child is not the main informant.
3. The child may not answer any questions at all, no matter how experienced the psychiatrist. Sometimes children or even teenagers who will not speak can be persuaded to draw or play a game.

The experience of *uninterrupted* time with total attention from a sympathetic adult will be new to many children.

Setting

There are great advantages in ensuring that diagnostic interviews with children of similar age are broadly comparable. The interview room should be arranged so that only the objects that are needed are in view. The clinician will chose toys and games to engage the child and aid the diagnostic process. Observation of a child is much more difficult in a room cluttered with toys. For the child aged 6 years or more it is usually preferable to spend most of the interview talking with him/her in the manner outlined in this chapter. With younger children and those with language or global delay there will need to be a greater reliance on non-verbal communication, and interaction will generally be easier if it occurs in a play situation.

With more mature children or adolescents the interview may often take more of the form of the adult psychiatric interview, but considerable modifications are still required since adults often come to the clinic because of their own concern over their problems. In contrast, the child or adolescent is generally referred because of someone else's concern.

General advice

1. Be non-judgemental.
2. But be prepared to specify limits: 'That's not what people do here.' 'I want you to stop doing that.'
3. Avoid long silences which can become persecutory, particularly for adolescents. Some can be engaged in a game; some will respond to 'I wonder if ...'.
4. Accept pictures if offered and keep them safely, as the child may ask about their offering on the next visit.
5. Do not speak in an artificial voice; children are quite tone responsive.
6. Do not rush in with direct interpretations.
7. Do not let the child take toys out of the room. 'Sorry, these toys belong to the hospital and there would be none for you to play with if you took one home every time.'
8. Warn about the end of the session five minutes before it finishes.

Common errors

1. Avoiding relevant but difficult topics in pursuit of a pleasant experience for the child.
2. Siding with the child instead of displaying a constructive neutrality.
3. Leading a suggestible child into inappropriate answers.
4. Building 'castles in the air' based on the nods of mute children.

Structure of interview

The structure and timing of the interview depend on context and need careful thought. A psychiatrist based in a community child and adolescent mental health service (CAMHS) will have to fit a considerable amount into a one-hour slot or conduct an extended assessment over several appointments. A psychiatrist working in a specialist service may have several hours or even an entire day to conduct an assessment. A single hour should be carefully structured with a focus on the presenting problem and its history, previous psychiatric history, medical and mental state examination. Other relevant history may have to be taken at the next available appointment.

Engagement

A short diagnostic family interview (10–15 minutes duration) provides a useful initial contact with the family. This can be followed by more formal history taking, an individual interview with the child, and psychometric assessment, as necessary. The clinician begins by explaining who s/he is (e.g. in the case of young children, 'I am a doctor who helps children and families with their problems') and the planned structure of the assessment. The family can then be asked to introduce themselves. Subsequently, it is helpful to ask the parents/carers if one may talk to the children first, and to engage the children individually on such (potentially) neutral topics as where they go to school and what that is like, whether they have friends, the names of their friends, what they like doing when at home or with friends, what they are good at. Having tried to engage all the children briefly in this way, it is important to explore with them why they think their parents decided that they should attend, preferably directing the question to a sibling of the referred child rather than to that child him/herself. The children are then encouraged to check with their parent(s) if their understanding regarding the reason for the appointment is correct. Exploration with the children regarding the reason for referral facilitates family communication around this issue, while at the same time clarifying the reasons for referral.

This joint time allows for the beginnings of an engagement with the children and family while observing family communication patterns, the emotional tone employed during communication (warm, critical, hostile, detached, understanding), and alliances between family members. Parents are generally pleased that time has been spent engaging their children in conversation and this time may act as a useful model for parents who have difficulty communicating with their child(ren).

Subsequent to the family interview, if co-workers are available, it is useful to split up so that one person can elicit a more formal history from the parents, while another can engage the child in an individual interview or more formal assessment. If siblings are present, they may be supervised by child-care staff (if available at the clinic) or an accompanying relative/family friend, or one parent may decide to monitor them while the other parent continues to participate in the assessment process. Information about the parent–child relationship can be gleaned from the parent(s) handling of the separation from the child and the child's response.

Children aged at least 6 years

Building rapport

Children will often be on the defensive, knowing that complaints have been made to the doctor about their behaviour. Therefore it is usually unwise to make any mention of the complaints at the beginning of the interview. The doctor should make it clear by the way s/he behaves towards the child that s/he is not acting as a judge or as someone who is going to correct or criticize. Rather, the aim is to show respect for the child as an individual and show interest in what s/he says and does.

If the child is expected to sit down for part of the interview, restless or uninhibited behaviour will be easier to observe. Allow the child to relax and talk freely, and assess the relationship s/he is able to form with the interviewer, the level and lability of his/her mood, his/her conversation, and any habitual mannerisms. In order to provide an adequate sample of behaviour, there should be about 15 minutes of unstructured conversation. The child should be encouraged to talk about recent events and activities, what sort of things s/he likes doing after school and at weekends, what s/he does with friends and families, the names of friends, the games s/he plays, what s/he enjoys and does not enjoy at school, etc. S/he may also be asked about hopes for the future, and what s/he wants to do when leaving school or grown up.

Respond with interest, concern, or enthusiasm, as appropriate. The interview must be geared to the child's age, intelligence, and interests. If the emotional responsiveness of the child is to be assessed adequately, it is necessary for the psychiatrist also to show a range of emotions (being more serious or concerned when asking about feelings of distress or worry, and more lively when responding to children's accounts of what interests or amuses them). Emotionally loaded topics should be pursued as they arise. The examiner's response should not block or lead away from expression of pathology or discomfort.

An approach to questioning

The child should then be questioned sympathetically about the specific information that should be elicited. Open questions are preferable but if the child finds it difficult to answer, then multiple choice questions can be useful. The interviewer could give specific examples of feelings or events. Indirect statements ('I knew a boy once about your age who...') may break the ice and allow the child to talk about difficult feelings. (If the child accepts this convention, there is no need to challenge it with statements such as 'This boy is you, isn't it?')

Ease off topics that seem too threatening, but consider returning to them later when the child is engaging more freely and appears more comfortable with the discussion. Does the child ever feel lonely, get into fights, get teased, or picked on? Is s/he picked on more than most other children?

Why does s/he think s/he is picked on? Similarly, the child should be asked how s/he gets on with brothers and sisters. If s/he gets into fights, does s/he like fighting? Are they 'real' fights or 'friendly' fights?

The child should be asked specifically about worries, ruminations, fears, unhappiness, bad dreams, and the sorts of things that make him/her feel angry. For example, s/he might be asked, 'Most people tend to worry about some things. What kind of things do you worry about? Do you ever lie awake at night worrying about things? Do you ever get nasty thoughts on your mind that you cannot get rid of? Do you ever get fed up? Miserable? Cry? Feel really unhappy? Are there things you are particularly afraid of? What about the dark? Spiders? Dogs? Monsters? Do you ever dream? What about bad dreams? Or have nightmares? What kind of things make you angry and annoyed?' Suicidal thoughts should be pursued where appropriate.

If anything positive should come up in answer to these questions, the psychiatrist should probe regarding the severity, frequency, and setting of the emotions (e.g. 'Do you ever feel so miserable that you want to go away and hide? Or that you want to run away? When was the last time that happened? How often do you feel like that? What sort of things make you fed up? Do you feel like that at home? At school?').

Children can be very suggestible and will sometimes produce answers that they think the doctor wants. However, the anxious or depressed child can usually be distinguished by the affective state when talking about worries, fears, feeling fed up, etc. Although it is important to ask the child systematically about these issues, it is also necessary for much of the interview to consist of neutral or cheerful topics. Note whether the child spontaneously mentions worries or extends answers on those topics beyond the questions.

Drawing tasks and cognitive tests

The child could be asked to draw a picture of someone or a house and everyone who lives in it, and encouraged to talk about it. This provides the opportunity to assess his/her natural skills, persistence, and distractibility, and also his/her attitudes and feelings, insofar as they are expressed in the drawing and what they say about the drawing. Handedness and fine motor skills can be assessed at the same time.

To assess attention span, persistence, and distractibility, children should be given some tasks within their ability but near to its limits. The drawing constitutes one task; in addition, they might be asked to give the days of the week forwards and backwards, and the months of the year, and also to do some simple arithmetic (such as serial 7s from 100, serial 3s from 30, addition and subtraction, or multiplication tables). This is one situation in the interview where the child is stressed; emotionally loaded discussion is another. Tics and involuntary movements are often at their most apparent when the child is under stress, and should also be noted throughout the interview.

Note that **tics** are rapid, stereotyped, repetitive, non-rhythmic, predictable, and purposeless contractions of functionally related muscle groups, which can usually be imitated or suppressed voluntarily for a time; **stereotypies** are voluntary, repeated, isolated, identical, predictable, and often rhythmic actions, in which whole areas of the body are involved; and **mannerisms** are odd, stylized embellishments of goal-directed movement. Notice also whether the level of activity is increased: **restlessness** is an inability to remain in the seat appropriately, while **fidgetiness** refers to squirming in the seat or movements of parts of the body but not the whole child.

Children aged below 6 years

A play setting is usually more appropriate for a child of 6 years or under; and it may sometimes be desirable to use a play interview with older children.

Games and toys should be chosen (1) to be suitable for the child's age, sex, and social background, (2) to provide an interaction with the interviewer, and (3) to encourage communication and imaginative play. The psychiatrist should become used to using a small range of toys (e.g. farm animals, colours, a doll's house with figures, plasticine). Imaginative games such as the squiggle game (making a drawing out of the child's squiggle and getting the child to do the same out of your squiggle), playing with family figures, etc., elicit a range of behaviour and emotions. It is better to allow the parents to accompany the child to the consulting room and then, after a while, and if the child is willing, the parents can be asked to leave the room to give the examiner an opportunity to interact with the child.

It is important to allow the child to become used to the situation before the examiner makes an approach. Initially, it may be useful simply to let the child explore the room and the toys while the doctor makes a friendly remark or two and responds to the child's approaches, but makes no approach directly. The speed with which the child may engage with the examiner will vary considerably. The play situation used to make an assessment and the manner in which the child is questioned should be suitable for his/her level of maturity. Young children cannot be expected to give descriptions of how they feel or to answer complex questions containing long words about abstract concepts. Nevertheless, many can explain what they do at home, who they play with, etc.

Scheme for description of mental state

General description

Appearance, manner, style of dress, any evidence of neglect; response to separation from parents, entering the interview room, and the doctor's attempts to make contact.

The child's adjustment to the situation

Apprehension, appropriate or excessive reserve, emerging confidence, friendliness, disruption, and age appropriateness. Topics of spontaneous conversation.

Motor activity

- amount of movement: reduced or increased
- coordination
- involuntary movements
- posturing

- rituals
- hyperventilation.

If any problems are noted, fuller neurological evaluation is needed.

Language
- hearing: sounds, speech
- comprehension
- speech/vocalization/babble:
  - spontaneity
  - quantity, rate, and rhythm (e.g. stuttering)
  - pattern of intonation and stress
  - articulation (e.g. dysarthria)
  - grammatical accuracy and complexity
  - specific abnormalities (e.g. echoing, stereotyped features, I–you reversals, with written example if appropriate)
- gesture: imitation/comprehension/use.

If any problems are noted, go to 'Assessment of children with developmental disorders', p. 53.

Social response to interviewer
- social responsiveness to examiner's manner and comments (e.g. praise, reward)
- rapport and eye contact: quality, quantity
- reciprocity and empathy
- social style (e.g. reserved, shy, expansive)
- disinhibited, cheeky, precocious, teasing
- negativistic, non-compliant, untruthful
- eager to please, pursuing secondary gain.

If any problems are noted, go to 'Assessment of children with developmental disorders', p. 53.

Affect
- emotional expressiveness and range
- happiness
- anxiety: free-floating, situational, or specific phobias
- panic attacks
- observable tension
- signs of autonomic disturbance
- tearfulness
- sadness, wretchedness, despair, apathy
- thoughts of suicide or running away
- shame, embarrassment, perplexity
- anger, aggressiveness
- irritability.

Thought content
- worries, fears
- preoccupations, obsessions, suspicions
- hopelessness, guilt
- low self-esteem, self-hatred

- fantasies or wishes:
  - spontaneously mentioned
  - evoked (e.g. three wishes)
- quality of ideation/play
- abnormal beliefs or experiences.

Cognition

- attention span/distractibility
- persistence
- curiosity
- orientation in time and space
- memory.

Attainment

Reading, spelling, and arithmetic are best assessed with standardized tests (e.g. Neale and Schonell for reading). If a formal assessment by a psychologist is not available, the child should be asked to read simple passages, to recall their gist, and to write a sentence about a previous event. The fluency, accuracy, and comprehension of reading are all important. This testing is even more necessary for children with disruptive behaviour or frustration in the classroom.

Standardized measures

An increasing number of rating scales for parents and teachers are available, and standardized structured or semi-structured interviews are sometimes used clinically. The advantages of explicit and formalized interviewing schemes are that they ensure systematic cover of key parts, and can provide standards of whether a problem is severe enough to be deviant. A corresponding disadvantage is that they cannot cover everything. The crucial aspect of an individual case may be uncommon or even unique. Standardized schemes may divert attention away from the individually significant to what is common. They need to be supplemented with the general clinical enquiry that is described here. Most symptoms in child psychiatry are on a continuum with normality. The judgement of what constitutes a disorder should be based not only on the levels of symptoms but also on an assessment of their impact on the child and the family.

Rating scales for parents and teachers are valuable as group tests, and sometimes for screening purposes. However, they are not yet sufficiently sensitive or specific for diagnosing an individual child. Rater effects, as well as the child's behaviour, will determine how they are completed.

Interviewer's subjective response to child: conclusion

Finally, an opinion should be expressed on whether (and how) the child's mental state departs from the expected in relation to age, IQ, sex, and social background.

Sources of information

Children are usually referred as a result of adult concern about their behaviour. Collateral information from several sources is even more important in child psychiatry than it is in adult psychiatry. One needs accounts of the child's behaviour and emotions at home, at school, or at playgroup, and as observed during the assessment.

The child is continually developing. Symptoms and behaviour problems change with developmental stages, as do emotional needs. Even more than with adults, the assessment of behaviour and mental state needs to focus particularly on the aspects relevant to the individual child's developmental stage.

Children's social and personal development is strongly influenced by the relationships formed at home and at school. The attitudes of adult carers and the quality of caring relationships need assessment as well as the child's development.

Interviewing parents

The history taking consists of two aspects: (a) obtaining information about events and behaviour; (b) recording expressed feelings, emotions, or attitudes concerning these events or the individuals participating in them. Because much of the interview is concerned with eliciting precise factual material, it is important to establish early on that the interviewer is interested in feelings as well as events. Care should be taken to encourage positive and negative attitudes to an equal extent. Where the informant's feelings are in doubt, questions such as 'Does this kind of thing ever cause difficulties in the home?' or 'Does that ever make you feel on edge?' are also useful, but should be used sparingly. In assessing the informant's feelings and emotions, attention should be paid to the way things are said as well as to what is said. Differences in the tone of voice, shown in the speed, pitch, and intensity of speech, can be important in the recognition of emotions. Particular attention should be paid to expressed criticism, hostility, and warmth, and to whom it is directed. Facial expressions and gestures should also be taken into account.

It is desirable, when possible, to see both the mother and the father. The child's relationship with the father is as important as that with the mother. It is better not to rely on a second-hand account of the father obtained from the mother or vice versa. An interview with two parents together will often provide a good opportunity to observe their relationship. If the parents are divorced or separated and the child spends time with each of them, it may be more appropriate to see the other parent on a separate occasion, as well as seeing any new significant adults in the family.

Presenting problem

The interview with the parents begins with an enquiry about the problems or difficulties which are the chief cause of concern. The parents should tell their story in their own words and then be asked if there are any other difficulties. **Recent examples** of the problems should always be obtained as well as the **frequency** of the behaviour, its **severity**, and the **context** of its occurrence (e.g. at school or when the child is away from home). The circumstances which **antecede or precipitate** the behaviour and those which **ameliorate or aggravate** the difficulties should always be noted. Determine the time of onset of the difficulties and go back to the point in the child's development when his/her behaviour or emotions first appeared unusual, abnormal, or a cause for concern. Were there stresses at that time?

This part of the interview gives a good opportunity to assess parental feelings and attitudes, and their beliefs about the problem; and these should be carefully described. In addition, the interviewer should find out what strategies have been used to deal with the problem, and how much success or failure they have had with each method. It is also useful at this point to find out what effect the symptom has had on the rest of the family. If appropriate, the interviewer should also enquire as to what led to their seeking help with regard to the child's problem and why help has been sought now rather than at any other time.

If delayed or unusual development is prominent, whether global or specific, refer to 'Assessment of children with developmental disorders', p. 53.

Systematic questioning

Review of other symptoms

Emotions

Are they happy or miserable? What makes them cry? Are they worried, depressed, suicidal, irritable, sulky? Do they have a temper? Exhibit fears and panics? Are there tears on getting to school, or even school refusal? Are they fussy? Are there specific things or situations that arouse fear? Are there any compulsions to do things? (NB: obsessions and compulsions in children are not necessarily accompanied by a subjective sense of resistance and may present as a handicapping ritual that cannot be explained.)

Antisocial trends

Are they disobedient? Destructive? Do they set fires? Tell lies? Steal? Are these problems only at home or outside? Do they happen when alone or with others? How are the problems dealt with? Has there been truancy or running away? Do they smoke, drink, sniff glue, or take drugs? Are they cruel to animals? Has there been any trouble with the police?

If the answer to any of these questions is 'yes', obtain details and enquire about the child's attitudes to discipline.

Activity and concentration

Are they overactive or restless? Will they stay still if expected to or are they always fidgety? How good is their concentration and what is the longest time they can concentrate on something interesting? Is there any change or loss of interest?

Eating, sleeping, and elimination

Are there eating difficulties at home or at school? Do they show food refusal or faddiness? Pica? Do they have sleeping difficulties: poor settling at night, waking in the night, nightmares? What are the sleeping arrangements? Is there enuresis: diurnal or nocturnal? Wetting when away from home? Have they ever been dry? Is there soiling or smearing? Have they ever been clean? Where is the lavatory? (Regularity of function is also a temperamental attribute.)

Current functioning
Typical day
A time budget helps to establish the context for children who are being assessed. In term time, who wakes up first? What happens? Who gets breakfast? How do the children behave first thing? How long do they take to get dressed? Who takes them to school? What are they like when they get home? What do they do then? How closely are they supervised? How do they behave during the evening meal; and when they are going to bed? What are the activities, and who provides care, during the school holidays? (NB: this enquiry is essentially to establish the framework; do not spend a long time on meticulous recording of exact details.)

Peer relationships
Although poor peer relationships are not a specific disorder, they are a good indicator of general adjustment. What are the names of any friends? What do they do together? How close are they? How long have they been friends? Do they visit each other's houses? Do other children reject or ignore? Does the child like to be with others or prefer to be alone? Are peer relationships within a group in which conduct and defiance issues are considered normal or desirable (e.g. a gang)?

Sibling relationships
How do they get on? Is the child closer to a particular sibling? How is this shown? Are there squabbles and with whom? Do they come to blows? Is there jealousy?

Relationships with adults
(This is also a convenient time to discover parental attitudes.) How does the child get on with mother/father? How is affection shown? Are they an easy child to get on with? How do they compare with other children? Whom do they take after and how? How do they get on with other adults? With teachers? Is there anyone they are particularly attached to? Does anyone help to look after them? What is it about them that parents find hardest to deal with or understand?

Family structure, family life, and relationships
Make note of appearance, manner, and mental state of parental informant(s).

Persons in home
Obtain a list. It may be helpful to draw a family tree. Ask about age, religion, occupation, education, and health of each person. Have the child's parents been married before? Are they adopted or fostered? Mother's pregnancies, including miscarriages and stillbirths. Make sure biological parents are identified. Get the same details about a parent or siblings who live away from home.

For important people outside the home
Establish what contact there is and the child's relationship (e.g. grandparents and parental siblings). Obtain a sketch of the parent's own childhood.

Parental relationship
How do the parents get on with each other? What things do they enjoy doing together? How do they spend evenings and weekends? To what extent does each parent participate in child care, discipline, and household tasks?

Parent–child interaction
What activities are done by parent and child jointly? Do they go out together? Play together? Help with homework? Help make things?

Child's participation in family activities
Does the child need help with dressing, feeding, etc.? Who helps? Does the child help with washing up, shopping, errands, etc.?

Family patterns of relationships
Are they closer to their mother or father? Who do they confide in? Father or mother? What attachments are there to other adults?

Rules at home
Do they have bedtime rules? Do they climb on furniture? Do they leave the house without saying where they are going, etc.? Are there restrictions on friends, staying out late, reading, or television? Who monitors the child's behaviour? Who tells the child off when discipline is needed? What method of punishment is used? Do they receive pocket money?

Family history of medical and mental health problems

A history of disorders in biological relatives needs to be taken carefully, because of the importance of genetic factors. For each first-degree relative, one should question to determine the presence or absence of any psychiatric disorders, psychiatric treatment, depression, suicide, language delay, difficulty in learning to read, enuresis, social oddness, alcoholism, epilepsy, and court appearances. Age of onset is helpful. For the more extended family, establish not only which members of the family, if any, have had mental problems, but their exact position in the family, and the other members who have not had problems. If there is a familial disorder, the pattern of transmission needs to be established.

Home circumstances

A home visit is not done routinely, but it can provide the best quality information and can often throw light on puzzling aspects of the history. Does the child live in a house or flat? How many rooms are there? Are there others in the home? What are the sleeping arrangements? Facilities (bath, lavatory, etc.)?

Other care arrangements
Does anyone else look after them: grandparents, baby-minder, neighbour after school, au pair, divorced parent at weekends, etc.?

Finances
What sources of finance are there? Are there any difficulties?

Neighbourhood
How long has the child lived there? Give a description of the area. Is it liked or disliked? Is there conflict with their neighbours? Is there any environmental threat (e.g. frequent assaults)?

Personal history

A general account of the art of eliciting a developmental history can be found in 'Assessment of children with developmental disorders', p. 53.

Pregnancy
Was it planned or not, and in what circumstances (e.g. adverse reaction of mother's own parents, abandoned by baby's father)? Were there complications such as pre-eclampsia or haemorrhage, or stresses such as infection, smoking, alcohol, drugs, or X-rays?

Delivery
Enquire about the place of birth (home or hospital), length of labour, presentation, mode of delivery, maturity, birth-weight, complications. Was resuscitation given: incubator or Special Care Baby Unit? Obtain details of the mother's health during and after pregnancy, including depression.

Neonatal period
Were there difficulties breathing or sucking? Cyanotic attacks? Convulsions? Jaundice? Floppiness? Infection? Were they kept in hospital longer than usual?

Feeding and sleep pattern in infancy
Were they breast or bottle fed? When were they weaned? Were there difficulties? Normal sleep pattern? Describe any difficulties.

Social development in infancy
Were they placid or active? Irritable? What was their response to mother? Did they cry a lot? What other attachments did they have?

Milestones
Useful stages to ask about include sitting unsupported, walking unaided, first word with meaning, and first two-word phrases. Comparison with siblings' development is helpful when exact stages are not remembered. Currently, do they speak as well as others of the same age, or do they have difficulty in understanding or producing speech, or in pronunciation, such as a lisp, baby talk, or stutter? If there are marked difficulties, see Table 3.1. Do they show clumsiness? Is there preference for a particular hand and foot? Do they have any twitches? Where? Head banging? Habits or rituals?

Bladder and bowel control
When were they dry by day and by night? (This is expected by the age of 5 years.) When did they have bowel control? (This is expected by the age of 4 years.) Were there any difficulties? Was training used? If so, how was it done? Who trained: child-minders, nurseries, playgroups? How did they respond?

Table 3.1 Scheme for current speech and language

1.	Imitation	Of housework etc.
2.	Inner language	Meaningful use of miniature objects, pretend play, drawing
3.	Comprehension of gesture	
4.	Comprehension of spoken language Hearing	Response to sounds; response to being called by name; reaction to loud noises; reaction to quiet meaningful sounds (mother's footsteps, noise of spoon in dish, food being prepared, door opening, rattle etc.); ever thought deaf?
	Listening and attention Understanding	Response to simple and complicated instructions with and without gesture (obtain details of examples)
5.	Vocalization and babble (non-speaking child)	
	Amount	
	Complexity	
	Quality	
	Social usage	Does s/he babble back to you?
6.	Language production	
	Mode	Gesture, pointing; taking by hand; speech
	Complexity	Syntactical and semantic; length of sentences; vocabulary; use of personal pronouns etc.
	Qualities	Echoing; stereotyped features; I–you confusion; made-up words; other oddities
	Amount Use of social communication	Asking for things; to comment or chat to and fro; in reply to questions; mute in certain situations
7.	Word-sound production	Any difficulties in pronunciation; consonants omitted or substituted; which ones; slurring; dysarthria; nasality Are speech defects consistent or variable?
8.	Phonation and volume of speech	
9.	Prosody	Pattern of stress and tonal variation in speech
10.	Rhythm Abnormalities	Stuttering; lack of cadence and inflection; coordination with breathing

Illness and allergies

Were they ever in hospital: inpatient, outpatient, clinic, operations, accidents? Have they had any serious illnesses: measles, meningitis, encephalitis, fits, or convulsions? Are they off school at all? Do they suffer from asthma, headaches, or stomach aches? How good is their sight and hearing? Do they suffer from fainting, fits, or absences? Any evidence of abnormal reactions to drugs or particular foods?

Separations

Have they ever been away from home without their parents or been separated while in hospital? Have they been apart from their parents for as long as 4 weeks? How were they looked after? What were the circumstances? How did they react?

Failures of care

Has there been any serious adversity in the past? Has caring been inadequate at any point (e.g. through illness, incapacity, or absence of a parent)? Has the child ever been maltreated (e.g. physical or sexual abuse)?

Schools

Which schools have they attended? How did they get on? Why were they changed? Has any teacher ever expressed concern to the parents? Has any statement of special education needs been made? Do they like the current school? Are progress reports satisfactory? Has the parent seen the child's teacher? (See 'Information from school and other sources outside the family', p. 52.)

Sex

Is there interest in the opposite sex? Has there yet been the development of menarche, body hair, or masturbation? Have they been instructed about sex, asked questions, or had any sexual experience? Is there any inappropriate sexual behaviour?

Strengths

What are the child's good qualities, abilities, and attractive attributes?

Temperamental or personality attributes

It is not easy to disentangle the child's premorbid characteristics from the present problems, but an attempt should be made. Some aspects of temperament are best shown in the response to new situations, new events, and new people, but attention should also be paid to the mode of functioning in routine situations.

Meeting new people

What is the child's behaviour with adults? With children? Do they approach strangers? Are they shy or clinging? How quickly do they adapt to someone new?

New situations

How do they react to new places, new gadgets, and new foods? Do they explore or hang back? How quick are they to adapt?

Emotional expression

How vigorous are they in expressing their feelings? Do they whimper or howl? Chuckle or roar with laughter? How happy/miserable were they before the present problems? How do they show their feelings?

Affection and relationships

Are they affectionate? Do they confide in anybody and if so, who? What friendships have they formed?

Sensitivity

How do they respond to a person or animal being hurt? What is their reaction if they have done something wrong?

Information from school and other sources outside the family

Parental consent should always be obtained to contact any agency other than the referrer and the family doctor. In medico-legal work, consent is needed to contact any agency other than the referrer. Permission to contact the school and other involved agencies can be requested when the first appointment is sent. If permission is not given for a key contact, such as that with the family doctor, it needs to be sought, with detailed discussion and explanation of its importance.

A teacher's account of the child's behaviour at school is indispensable. Ask for information about:

- attendance
- academic strengths and weaknesses
- non-academic skills (e.g. art, music, woodwork, sports)
- behaviour in the classroom and playground
- social relationships with teachers and peers
- any other observations of importance.

For preschool children, a report along the same lines from a nursery or playgroup leader is of similar importance. It can be helpful to have this information available at the first assessment.

It is good practice to explain to the family that a letter will be sent to the family doctor after the assessment and a request made to obtain old medical records etc. The family doctor frequently possesses further essential information. In medico-legal work, the final report will be sent only to the referrer, who will then distribute it to the appropriate parties.

Psychological testing will usually be an important part of the systematic assessment of a child and will usually provide quantified information from behaviour and performance in a rigorously controlled setting. Such an assessment needs to be interpreted in the light of the validity of the test and the nature of the problem. A low test score from an uncooperative child should not necessarily be taken as implying a limitation of intellectual potential. A normal or high IQ score in a child with problems in everyday learning does not necessarily entail a non-cognitive explanation; there may be impairment in aspects of cognition that are not assessed by the tests used. If the clinical appraisal of cognitive functioning is discrepant with the psychometric evaluation, further enquiry is needed to find out why.

Synthesizing different sources

Evidence often conflicts. There is no single rule for how to resolve disagreements; clinical judgement is required.

When there is disagreement, first evaluate whether any of the sources is likely to be unreliable. Is the mother depressed and exaggerating psychopathology, or fearful of the consequences of the assessment and suppressing problems? Have the parents read accounts of disorders such as autism and presented a 'textbook' account? Does a teacher have insufficient acquaintance with the child to be accurate?

Next, consider whether disagreement comes from varying standards about what is expected from a child. Care givers vary greatly in their beliefs about the degree of deviance that is required before they decide that a problem is present. It will not be enough to establish that a parent considers, for example, that their child is hyperactive. Rather, detailed enquiry will be needed to establish actual behaviours such as the length of time for which the child engages in constructive activities, and the time for which they can remain still in a situation where this is expected. Parents are often much better at recall of details of behaviour than at judgement of what is the range of normality, and so apparent disagreements may disappear on close enquiry.

For some problems, priority should be given to one source of information. Children describe their depressed feelings more frequently than adults recognize them. Therefore, the parental account may be insensitive, and the rule is often adopted that the symptom of depression is present if *any* informant gives a clear account of a marked problem in the child. In contrast, antisocial conduct may be denied by the child, especially if the parents are present, so that the parental account is often more sensitive.

For many problems, accounts may differ because the child is different in different situations. This specificity to context is in itself important diagnostic information. For example, hyperactivity that is pervasive across all sources of information is more likely to be based on neurodevelopmental dysfunction than the same behaviour that is seen only in one setting, such as school.

Finally, if doubt persists after careful enquiry and consideration of possible reasons, the best way of resolving disagreements is for the psychiatrist to make observations directly in the natural settings.

Assessment of children with developmental disorders

It is usually most convenient to begin with a chronological account of development. However, rather than go immediately to questions of pregnancy and delivery, it may be preferable to start by asking the parents when they first became concerned that something might be not quite right with the child's development, and what it was that aroused their concern at the time. Particularly with a first child, the parents' concern may have been aroused long after the child first showed delays or distortions in development. It is helpful to enquire whether, with hindsight, the parents think that all was well before they first became concerned and, if not, what it was that might have been abnormal. Having established the time and nature of those first indications of concern, it is generally easiest to go back to the time of pregnancy and work forwards systematically up to the present time. Most parents do not remember at all accurately when milestones occurred if they were within the normal range, but they are more likely to recall them if they were delayed. It is helpful to focus on that aspect first before going on to tie down the time more exactly. When seeking to date milestones, reference should be made to familiar landmarks rather than to ages as such. It might be appropriate, for example, to ask whether the child was walking on his first birthday, or when they moved house, or at the time of his first Christmas, or when the second child was born.

Particular attention needs to be paid to the developmental aspects of play, socialization, and language. With respect to the milestones of language, it is crucial to be quite specific about what is being asked. Parents are very inclined to interpret all manner of sounds as speech, and especially as 'mama' and 'dada'. Consequently, it may be wise to ask very focused questions such as: 'When did he first use simple words with meaning, that is words other than mama and dada?' ; 'What were his first words?'; 'How did he show that he knew their meaning?'. In addition to the first use of single words, it is important to ask about babble, the use of two- or three-word phrases, the use of pointing, gesture, or mime, following instructions, and immediate or delayed echoing. It is helpful to identify some occasions that the parents remember reasonably clearly and then to focus on what the child was like at that time. In doing so, an attempt should be made to determine what the child was like at about 2 years, 30 months, 3 years, and 4 years.

Few parents think of socialization in terms of milestones or indeed in terms of specific behaviours. As a result, although the topic may be introduced by some general question such as 'How affectionate was he as a toddler?', it will always be necessary to proceed with a series of focused questions directed at eliciting information in key aspects of social relationships and social responsiveness at particular ages. Thus, for the 6–12 month age period, it would be necessary to ask whether the child turned to look the parents directly in the face when they spoke to him/her, whether s/he put up his arms to be lifted, whether s/he nestled close when held, whether s/he protested when left, whether s/he laughed and chortled in response to parental overtures, whether s/he was comforted by being picked up and cuddled, and whether s/he was wary of strangers. Similarly with toddlers, questions should be asked about whether the child greeted a parent coming home, whether s/he sought to be cuddled when upset or hurt ('Did he come to you or did you have to go to him?'), whether s/he differentiated between parents and others to whom s/he went for comfort, whether s/he showed separation anxiety, and whether s/he could be playful and enter into the spirit of to-and-fro in a teasing or make-believing game.

Precise questions are required to elicit an adequate account of the child's play at particular ages. Thus, to determine whether play was normal at age 2 years, the clinician should ask about the child's use of toys and other objects. Did s/he recognize the appropriate use of miniature toys, such as pushing toy cars along the floor making car noises, or rather did s/he tend to spin the wheels, feel the texture of the paint, or listen to the sound of a wind-up car? Was there any pretend play, such as the use of toy tea sets, dolls, etc.? Would the pretend play vary from day to day and would the pretend element be used to create any sort of sequence of story (e.g. with the toy cars racing each other, being parked in the garage, or being used to go to Granny's home)?

Having obtained a history of the development of play, social interaction, and language, with special reference to the first 5 years, it is necessary to obtain a comparably specific account of the child's **current behaviour** in these areas of functioning. Before proceeding to direct questioning on particular features, it is helpful to gain an overall picture of the child's activities by asking how s/he spends his time on return from school or at a weekend. Such a description usually provides a life-like portrayal of the bleakness or richness of the child's inner and outer world, and focuses attention on the activities and experiences to be asked about in greater detail. For adequate evaluation to be possible, the specific questioning should be based on a systematic scheme that ensures that each of the crucial areas is covered, as set out in Tables 3.1–3.3.

Table 3.2 Scheme for current social interaction

1.	Differentiation between people	Shown by different responses to mother, father, stranger, etc.
2.	Selective attachment	
	Source of security or comfort	To whom does s/he go when hurt?
	Greeting	E.g. parent returning from work
	Separation anxiety	
3.	Social overtures	
	Frequency and circumstances	
	Appropriateness to the situation	
	Quality	Visual gaze, facial expression; enthusiasm
4.	Social responses	
	Frequency and circumstances	
	Quality	Eye-to-eye gaze, facial expression; emotions
	Reciprocity	To-and-fro dialogue
5.	Social play	
	Playfulness	
	Spontaneous imitation	
	Cooperation and reciprocity, sharing	
	Emotional expression	
	Pleasure in the other person	
	Humour	
	Social excitement	

Table 3.3 Scheme for current play

1.	Social aspects	See Table 3.1
2.	Cognitive level	
	Curiosity	
	Understanding how things work	
	Complexity	Puzzles; drawing; rule-following; inventiveness
	Imagination	Pretend play; creativity; spontaneity; telling stories
3.	Content, type, and quality	
	Initiation	
	Variable or stereotyped	
	Unusual preoccupations	
	Unusual object attachments	
	Rituals and routines	
	Resistance to change	
	Stereotyped movements	
	Interest in unusual aspects of people or objects	
4.	Attention	
	Orientation to a new situation and a new toy	
	Distractibility to extraneous stimuli	
	Length of time playing with each toy, and frequency of change of activity	
	Persistence vs leaving play activities unfinished	
	Acceptance of, and persistence with, toys or activities introduced by the examiner	

The mental state examination

This chapter deals with the mental state examination of adults and also includes special points concerning examination of the elderly. Special aspects of the examination (neuropsychiatric assessment of both adults and children; examination of those with epilepsy or catatonia, or who are mute or in a stupor) are considered in Chapter 5.

The mental state of adults

The mental state examination elicits a snapshot of a patient's behavioural and psychological functioning. Its description should record information gained by examination during the interview as well as other relevant observations (e.g. those made elsewhere in the clinic or hospital). There are three aspects to interviewing: obtaining information, observing the patient in a two-person interaction, and giving support.

One should always try to put the patient at ease, as only too frequently patients fail to mention crucial information through fear or anxiety. By doing this, benefits above and beyond the collection of clinical information can be achieved. For example, a well-conducted interview gives a depressed or anxious patient an opportunity to explain his/her problems to a doctor who, by asking about each symptom suffered, may be perceived to 'understand'. Therefore, the mental state examination provides the interviewer with an opportunity to develop a therapeutic relationship further, and to offer empathy and support.

When describing the mental state of a patient, it is rarely useful to employ the terms 'normal' or 'abnormal' since these terms convey little. Instead, a description of the signs and symptoms elicited should be recorded under the headings listed in this chapter. This will enable others to form clinical judgements as to the significance of the information gathered, and will also be very useful for future reference.

Appearance and general behaviour

Few doctors are gifted with the descriptive talent of Charles Dickens, but a decent portrayal of a patient's appearance and behaviour is within the abilities of most. One should aim to give as complete, accurate, and life-like a description as possible of how the patient appears and what can be observed in his/her behaviour.

Describe the patient's physical characteristics and his/her general behaviour. Is it appropriate, bizarre, incongruous, or agitated? Consider his/her personal self-care (cleanliness in general, hair, cosmetics, dress), eating, sleep, posture, and facial expression (depressed, elated, or anxious). Is s/he relaxed or tense and restless; slow, hesitant, or repetitive? How does s/he behave towards other patients, doctors, and nursing staff? Is s/he warm and open, or guarded, hostile, and threatening? Does s/he show good eye contact? Is s/he distractible or unresponsive? Does s/he appear frightened or frightening? Does s/he respond abnormally to external events? Can his/her attention be held and diverted?

Does s/he appear over-emotional (is s/he dancing and singing, or withdrawn, tearful, and sullen; wringing hands with anxiety or relaxed; preoccupied and perplexed, or does s/he show little emotional expression)? Does s/he appear to be responding to hallucinations? Does his/her behaviour suggest that s/he is disorientated? Specify orientation if doubtful. Do his/her movements, comportments, and dispositions have an apparent purpose or meaning? Describe any motor abnormalities such as gestures, grimaces, tics, mannerisms, stereotypes, waxy flexibility, slowness, tremor, and rigidity. Is there much or little activity? Does it vary during the day? Is it spontaneous, or how is it provoked? If s/he is inactive, does s/he resist passive movements, obey commands, or indicate awareness at all? A detailed account of the appearance and behaviour of catatonic, mute, or stuporose patients is especially valuable (these presentations are considered in detail in Chapter 5).

Speech

The form of the patient's utterances, rather than their content, is considered here. Does s/he say much or little, speak loudly or quietly, talk spontaneously or only in answer, slowly or quickly, hesitantly or promptly, to the point or wide of it, coherently, anxiously, discursively, loosely with interruptions, with sudden silences, with frequent changes of topic? Does s/he comment appropriately on events and things at hand, or does s/he use strange words or syntax, rhymes, puns, clang associations? How does the form of his/her talk vary with its subject? Is s/he monotonous or lyrical?

Verbatim samples of talk should be recorded so as to demonstrate any abnormalities such as flight of ideas, thought block, derailments of thought, incoherence or drivelling, reiterations, perseveration, neologisms, paraphasias, etc. Samples of what the patient actually said are more useful than your opinion as to whether, for example, s/he employed neologisms. Attach or include in the notes any examples of the patient's writing which appear abnormal.

Mood

The patient's appearance, motility, posture, and general behaviour, as already described, may give some indication of his/her mood. In addition, his/her answers to questions such as 'How do you feel in yourself?', 'What is your mood?', 'How about your spirits?', or similar enquiries, should be recorded. Whenever depressive mood is suspected, specific enquiry should be made about the following: tearfulness, diurnal variation of mood, initial and middle insomnia, early morning wakening. Consider any suicidal ideas or plans, his/her attitude to the future, hopelessness, self-esteem, worthlessness, and guilt. Note any loss of appetite, weight, energy, motivation or libido, or constipation. Many variations of mood may be present, not merely happiness or sadness (e.g. such states as anxiety, fear, suspicion, or perplexity). Observe the constancy of the mood during the interview, those influences which change it, and the appropriateness of the patient's apparent emotional state to what s/he says. Note evidence of flatness, reactivity, or lability of affect, and specify any indications that the patient is concealing his/her true feelings.

Symptoms and behaviours associated with mania (elevated mood, little need for sleep or food, excessive energy, reckless behaviour, initiation of multiple tasks without completion, distractibility) and anxiety (tremor, dry mouth, butterflies, blurred vision, sweating) should also be evaluated and recorded here.

Thought content

The content of the patient's thoughts, rather than their form, is considered here. The patient's answers to questions such as 'What do you see as your main worries?' should be summarized. Are there any morbid thoughts, anxieties, or preoccupations regarding his/her past, present, and future? Do worries interfere with concentration or sleep? Are there any phobias or obsessional ruminations, compulsions, or rituals?

Abnormal thoughts should be comprehensively described and their precipitants, mode of onset, duration, intrusiveness, frequency, congruity with mood, fixity, and effect upon the patient's functioning noted. The description given should be full enough to allow future readers to make their own decision as to whether the patient suffered from, for example, a phobia, obsessional rumination/compulsion, overvalued idea, idea of reference, or delusion (including delusions of passivity and thought possession), all of which should be recorded within this section.

This section should always include an evaluation of any thoughts of harm towards self or others. Should such thoughts be admitted, a detailed account of the patient's intent should be recorded, including the onset, frequency, planning, preparation, and desire to harm. The patient should also be asked whether s/he believes that s/he is capable of realizing these thoughts, and if there are any factors that are preventing him/her from completing the act.

Abnormal beliefs and interpretations of events

Specify the content, mode of onset, degree of fixity, pre-occupation, and distress of any unusual or abnormal beliefs.
1. In relation to the environment (e.g. ideas of reference, misinterpretations, or delusions); beliefs that s/he is being persecuted, that s/he is being treated in a special way, or is the subject of an experiment.
2. In relation to the body (e.g. ideas or delusions of bodily change).
3. In relation to the self (e.g. delusions of passivity, influence, thought reading, or intrusion).

Abnormal experiences

Abnormalities in perception should be recorded here.
1. Environment: hallucinations or illusions (auditory, visual, olfactory, gustatory, or tactile) as well as feelings of familiarity or unfamiliarity, derealization, or *déjà vu*.
2. Body: feelings of deadness, pain, or other alterations of bodily sensation; somatic hallucinations.
3. Self: depersonalization; awareness of disturbance in mechanism of thinking, blocking, retardation, autochthonous ideas, etc.

The source, content, vividness, reality, duration, and other characteristics of these experiences should be recorded, together with the time of occurrence (e.g. at night, when alone, when falling asleep, or on awakening). Ascertain exacerbating or ameliorating factors as well as the patient's insight into the cause, in addition to the significance and emotional impact, of any perceptual abnormality.

The cognitive state

This should be briefly assessed in every patient and related to his/her premorbid intelligence (see Chapter 5, 'Mental state examination', p. 69). For younger patients, who are not suspected of cerebral organic disease, the following tests for orientation, attention, concentration, and memory should be administered. For older patients, see 'The elderly', p. 64. When cognitive impairment or cerebral disease is suspected, additional tests will need to be given from the schema for further examination of patients with suspected organic cerebral disease (see Chapter 5, 'Mental state examination', p. 69).

Orientation

If there is any reason to doubt the patient's orientation, record the patient's answers to questions about his/her own name and identity, the place where s/he is, the time of day, and the date.

Attention and concentration

Is his/her attention easily aroused and sustained? Does s/he concentrate? Is s/he easily distracted? To test his/her concentration and attention, ask him/her to tell the days or the months in reverse order, or to do simple arithmetical problems requiring 'carrying over' (e.g. 112–25) or subtraction of serial 7s from 100 (give answers and time taken). Give digits to repeat forwards, and then others to repeat backwards (delivered evenly and at one-second intervals), and record how many s/he can reproduce in each direction.

Memory

In all cases memory should be assessed by comparing the patient's account of his/her life with that given by others, and by examining his/her account for intrinsic evidence of gaps or inconsistencies. Special attention should be paid to memory for recent events, such as those of his/her admission to hospital and happenings in the ward since then. However, questions such as 'What did you have for breakfast?' are only useful if you know the answer yourself. Where there is selective impairment of memory for special incidents, periods, or recent or remote happenings, this should be recorded in detail, and the patient's attitude to his/her forgetfulness and the things forgotten particularly investigated. Record any evidence of confabulation or false memories. If the patient confabulates, is this spontaneous or in response to suggestion only? Retrograde and anterograde amnesia must be specified in detail in relation to head injury or epileptic phenomena.

Intelligence

The patient's expected intelligence should be gauged from his/her history, general knowledge, and educational and occupational record. Where this is unknown, simple tests for general information and grasp should be given, and an assessment made of his/her experience and interests. An indirect measure of intelligence may also be obtained from assessing the patient's scholastic achievements by testing his/her reading, spelling, and arithmetical abilities. A more objective measure can be obtained by using the Mill Hill and Progressive Matrices Tests from which an intelligence quotient (IQ) can be derived. Disorder should be suspected if a discrepancy is found between the results of these tests and the level of intelligence anticipated by assessing the patient's literacy and numeracy, or if performance measures are markedly inferior to verbal measures.

Patient's appraisal of illness, difficulties, and prospects

What is the patient's attitude to his/her present state? Does s/he regard it as an illness, as 'physical', 'mental', or 'nervous', or as needing treatment? What does s/he attribute it to? Is s/he aware of any mistakes s/he made spontaneously or in response to tests? How does s/he regard them and other details of his/her condition? How does s/he regard previous experiences, mental illnesses, etc.? Can s/he appreciate possible connections between his/her illness and stressful life situations, spontaneously or when suggested? Are his/her attitudes constructive or unconstructive, realistic or unrealistic? Is his/her judgement good when discussing financial or domestic problems etc.? What does s/he propose to do when s/he has left the hospital or clinic? What is his/her attitude to supervision and care?

The interviewer's reaction to the patient

If it is appropriate, a brief account may be given of the way in which the interviewer is affected by the patient's behaviour. Did the patient arouse sympathy, concern, sadness, anxiety, irritation, frustration, impatience, or anger?

The elderly

Most older people have no objections to cognitive assessment when it is introduced with tact. It is helpful to start off by asking whether the patient has experienced any problems with memory and concentration (and, if so, whether this has bothered them and what sort of things they find that they forget). After this, the cognitive assessment may make more sense. A useful preamble is as follows: 'I am going to ask a few questions about memory and concentration. Some of these may seem very easy and others might be quite difficult, but we need to ask everyone the same questions.'

Some patients with dementia are unwilling to undergo formal testing and respond with irritation, unexplained refusal, or bland replies such as 'I don't pay attention to that sort of thing'. Such replies may be an attempt to camouflage an impairment and should be handled with tact. A reliable collateral history is invaluable in these situations.

Where the patient agrees to formal testing, a short cognitive screening test such as the Mini-Mental State Examination (MMSE) or the Abbreviated Mental Test (AMT) can be used. The MMSE can give an approximate idea of the severity of impairment in dementia, while a high score may provide evidence against substantial cognitive impairment. It may also be helpful in future assessments to have an idea of prior function and, therefore, it is important that previous assessments are obtained, wherever possible, so as to put any current score in context.

Interpreting the scores on cognitive impairment scales

Some cognitive impairment scales are found in Appendix 2. It is vital to take previous education, levels of literacy, and sensory deficits into account when interpreting scores from these screening tests. For example, someone with high educational attainment may have clinically evident dementia and still achieve a maximum score on the MMSE. Unfortunately, both screening tests have poor cross-cultural validity and results should be interpreted with appropriate caution.

Scores of 6 or below on the AMT indicate possible dementia and the need for a more formal assessment (unless the test is being used in primary care to assess progress in a patient with known dementia).

The MMSE was developed at Johns Hopkins University for use in neurological patients but has since been validated in a wide variety of settings. A score of 23 or less is indicative of 'dementia'. The MMSE is sensitive to the effects of age, educational background, and socio-economic status. For patients aged over 70 years, who left school before 15, the cut-point should be reduced by three points.

Cognitive screening tests such as the MMSE provide relatively little information concerning specific cognitive deficits such as impairment of memory or frontal lobe function and the ACE is more informative in this regard. If cognitive impairment is suspected, a neuropsychiatric assessment should be carried out as outlined in Chapter 5.

Mood state

Some elderly patients with profound depression deny depressed mood, but show other prominent symptoms such as anxiety, somatic or dissociative symptoms, or cognitive impairment.

Psychotic and behavioural problems

These can be best elicited from an informant.

Physical examination

Many elderly patients suffer from concurrent physical illness, and a thorough physical examination should always be carried out. Special attention should be given to any signs of physical trauma, possibly occurring as a result of abuse.

Neuropsychiatric assessment

History

A good history is the most valuable diagnostic tool in neuropsychiatry. The history should elicit the physical and psychological symptoms and, most importantly, give a clear chronology of how these developed. Examination should be considered confirmatory. It is useful to be able to tailor the examination to the differential diagnosis emerging from the history.

Presenting complaint

When was change first noticed? Who noticed it first? Did it come on suddenly or gradually? Over hours, days, weeks? When was help first sought? What did the patient understand the symptoms meant? Aggravating or relieving factors? In a complex history, a useful question may be 'When were you last really well?' or 'How far back would you have to go to say you had no problems of this kind?'. Collateral history from an informant is crucial in confirming onset and course of the disorder, particularly when there is suspicion of cognitive impairment either at the time of initial presentation or at the time of examination (see Table 5.1). This may mean discussion with family, friends, and work colleagues, as well as professional staff who have had contact with the patient. If this is not possible, it should be clearly recorded that the assessment is provisional and collateral is still needed.

Family history

History of specific disorders: seizures, movement disorders, cerebrovascular disease. History of dementia and, if so, age of onset. Family history of early onset dementias may be much more significant than dementia complicating late life.

Personal history
- Obstetric complications?
- Delayed walking/talking or other milestones?
- Any learning difficulties?
- Educational attainment?
- Sick child, frequent attendances at doctor or hospital?

Table 5.1 Time course and diagnosis of neuropsychiatric disorder

Rapid decline and complete recovery	Transient ischaemic attack, epilepsy, transient global amnesia, relapsing/remitting multiple sclerosis
Slow steady decline	Alzheimer's disease, Huntington's disease, Parkinson's disease, normal pressure hydrocephalus
Rapid steady decline	Encephalitis, brain tumour, raised intracranial pressure, cerebral abscess, atypical dementia
Stepwise deterioration	Vascular dementia, progressive multiple sclerosis
Diurnal variation	Myasthenia gravis
Static condition	Autism, Asperger's syndrome, cerebral palsy

- Performance decline at work?
- Any occupational hazards (e.g. lead or solvents)?
- Amount, type, frequency, mode of administration (e.g. intravenous) of recreational drugs consumed, especially alcohol; pattern of consumption over time.

Previous medical history
- Any childhood infections, fits?
- Any head injury? If so, degree of amnesia before and after and any loss of consciousness (check examiner and patient share understanding of this term—loss of awareness).
- Ever seen a neurologist or physician?

Prescribed medications
- Names, duration, benefits if any. Why prescribed?
- Has the patient suffered any side effects?
- History of episodes of toxicity.

Social history
- Carers, nature of care needed, attitude to carers.
- Adaptations of home, when and how arranged? Level of statutory benefits received?
- Children, ages, awareness of diagnoses (especially relevant to genetic conditions).

Level of function
Typical day. Ability to self-care. Toilet, feeding, transferring to chair/bed, general mobility. Best day? Worst day?

Forensic history
History of offending and attitude to offending may be particularly important for patients with dysexecutive syndromes and/or head injuries.

Mental state examination

The mental state examination will comprise some formal cognitive tests but the overall examination is continuous during the interview. Valuable time is saved observing the patient's gait, spontaneity, social manner, language use, and response to environment, as the interview is proceeding. If cognitive impairment seems present, move to a full cognitive examination rather than struggle to obtain the history. If there is an apparent decreased level of consciousness, use the Glasgow Coma Scale (best verbal and motor responses, and pupillary reflex) to record this.

Cognitive examination
Orientation
Disorientation is a key indication of cerebral dysfunction, reflecting alterations in the level of consciousness. Time disorientation is regarded as the hallmark of acute organic reactions.

- Time/place/person: does the patient know who they are, where they are, and what the date is? Impairment of orientation to self is rare except in very advanced dementia or non-organic syndromes.

Attention and concentration
These test alertness and the capacity to control information processing in the brain. Along with tests for orientation, these are a means of evaluating the patient's level of conscious awareness.
- Reciting backwards: for example, give reverse days of the week or spell WORLD backwards.
- Serial 7s: counting down from 100 in subtractions of 7.
- Digit span recall—forwards and backwards: remember to deliver each digit in a monotone, one second apart (average, seven forward).

Language
Dysarthria, a difficulty in the mechanical production of speech, should be assessed before **dysphasia**, which is the cortical partial failure of language function. **Receptive dysphasia** can be detected by asking the patient to point to named objects in the environment, or to respond to a short series of verbal commands. You can test for **expressive dysphasia** by asking the patient to name everyday objects **(nominal dysphasia)** or write a sentence of his/her own choice. Do not forget to check handedness as 95 per cent of right-handers and the majority of left-handers have relative language dominance in the left hemisphere.
- Repetition
  - 'West Register Street' and 'no ifs, ands, or buts'.

This tests for dysarthria and the intactness of the connections between the input and output of speech. Minor errors may be common in non-native speakers. If in doubt, repeat, with a different phrase.
- Comprehension
  - Response to simple instructions:
    — Point correctly on command (e.g. surrounding objects).
    — Carry out simple orders on request (e.g. pick up an object, show tongue).
  - Response to complex instructions:
    — Tear paper into three pieces (Marie's three-paper test).
    — Can you point to the window after tapping the desk?
- Word finding
  - Name both common and uncommon objects (e.g. parts of a wrist watch and other objects in the room). Describe a picture.

This tests for nominal dysphasia (the reduced capacity to retrieve words used in everyday speech), which may be the only language disturbance. Note circumlocutions used to cover this deficit.
- Reading
  - Observe for content errors (also dysarthria and dysprosody).
- Writing
  - Test ability to write spontaneously and examine written productions for substitutions, perseverations, spelling errors, and letter reversals. Note that asking a patient to write something about what they have just read (e.g. a news item) also further tests their comprehension.

Memory

Amnesia (acquired memory dysfunction) is an abnormality of registering, storing, recalling, or recognizing information and events. **Focal amnestic states** can occur with relative preservation of other cognitive functions, which contrasts with **diffuse amnesic states**. All are qualitatively different from **psychogenic amnesias**. Memory failure is a particularly sensitive indicator of cerebral dysfunction. Your patient may have deficits in explicit memory, with difficulty in conscious recollection, yet retain implicit (procedural/skills) knowledge. For example, they may be able to find their way around familiar surroundings but be unable to recollect (describe) their route.

- Immediate memory span (or 'ultra-short-term memory')
  - Digit repetition (tested previously)
- Recent events
  - Recall of the temporal sequence of events (e.g. the events of the interview so far)
- New learning
- Name and address
  - Ask for immediate reproduction (testing **registration**) and record the answer verbatim (repeat if necessary). If one or more mistakes are made, the entire name and address should be provided again.
  - Test **retrieval** 3–5 minutes later after interposing other cognitive tests, and again record the answer verbatim.
- Recall (paired association): free and cued
  - Give patient a list of six to ten paired items (e.g. colour—blue, flower—daffodil, etc.) or use a simpler test of three-word recall, with each word being categorically different (e.g. car, river, monkey).

Giving verbal cues when spontaneous recall fails tests storage. A retrieval deficit is suggested if the patient's performance improves. Information processing is also being tested, as thinking of semantic links facilitates recall. These tests are especially valuable with anxious or disturbed patients.

- Sentence repetition
  - Ask the patient to repeat a sentence appropriate to their intellectual level, e.g.
    — 'Yesterday we went for a ride in our car along the road that crosses the bridge.'
    — 'The aeroplane made a careful landing in the space that had been prepared for it.'
    — 'The redheaded woodpeckers made a terrible fuss as they tried to drive the young away from the nest.'
    — 'One thing a nation needs to become rich and great is a large secure supply of wood.' (the Babcock sentence)

Test the number of repetitions necessary for accurate reproduction. (Three repetitions of a sentence such as this should allow word-perfect reproduction in most people of normal intelligence under 40.)

- General information
  - Semantic (conceptual) memory (e.g. names of key personalities, well-known dates, places, and events, both distant and current).
  - Episodic (personal) memory: matters unique to the individual (e.g. name of examiner, what the examiner has asked since the interview began).

- Non-verbal memory should be assessed by asking the patient to
reproduce a simple figure, such as a cross or a clock face showing
a specific time, after a 5-minute interval. Initial copying of the figure
tests **constructional praxis** (described in this section) as well as
registration.

Apraxia

Apraxia is the inability to perform a volitional act even though the peripheral
motor system and sensorium are intact. It is rarely seen without dysphasia,
except in the case of constructional dyspraxia:

- ability to imitate postures and make-believe movements (e.g. wave
goodbye)
- ability to perform a complex coordinated sequence of actions (e.g. fold
a letter and put it in an envelope).

Ideomotor apraxia is the inability to carry out simple coordinated movement
sequences on command, despite being able to carry out these actions spontaneously. It is associated with damage to the inferior parietal dominant hemisphere in right-handed patients. **Ideational apraxia** is the inability to carry out
a planned, complex coordinated sequence, despite demonstrating an ability to
carry out each individual component; it is rare and has been thought to be seen
in callosal lesions, extensive left hemisphere lesions, and in advanced dementia. **Constructional apraxia** has been tested by the drawing already mentioned.
Though not very well lateralized, it suggests right hemisphere dysfunction.
Dressing apraxia (said to be a non-dominant parietal lobe problem) is evident
from the informant or by asking the patient to dress. **Gait apraxia** is assessed by
the tandem gait test (see 'Neurological examination', p. 74).

Agnosias

Agnosias are relatively rare and complex disorders of perceptual recognition. The individual is unable to understand the significance of sensory
stimuli even though the sensory pathways and sensorium are intact. All
modalities may be affected but visuospatial problems are more common.

Visuospatial function

Tests are as follows.

- distance estimation between objects: tests proportions
- copy a diagram: tests constructional ability
- freehand drawing (e.g. drawing a clock face with numbers)
- describe an object and explain what it is.

Visuospatial agnosia (broadly synonymous with constructional apraxia)
and **hemineglect** will be shown by omissions in images copied. **Visual
object agnosia** (visual recognition failure) is present when the patient fails
to identify objects by sight and cannot name them, i.e. they are unable to
grasp the meaning of the object purely by looking at it (but can through
other senses). **Astereognosia** is the failure to identify three-dimensional
form and is tested by placing a familiar object (e.g. a key) in the patient's
hand. **Agraphaesthesia** is detected by tracing numbers on the palms with a
retracted ball-pen, which the patient then fails to recognize.

    Anosognosia is the term used to refer to some patients' inability to per-
ceive their own disability. It is seen in right-hemisphere stroke and can be
particularly disabling and resistant to rehabilitation.

Frontal lobe function

Evidence of frontal lobe damage would have been suggested by a history of behavioural disturbance, personality change, and 'executive dysfunction' (e.g. disturbance to planning and monitoring goal-directed behaviours). Other symptoms can include apathy, hyperorality (including overeating), and incontinence. Tests are as follows:

- Verbal fluency: ability to generate categorical lists, e.g. words beginning with the letter F (FAS test: >10 words per letter in 1 minute is expected).
- Motor sequencing (Luria's fist–edge–palm test): this should be assessed by first demonstrating the sequence to the patient and then asking him/her to copy and then continue the imitation (after the examiner has stopped) for at least 30 seconds. Remember to vary the sequence between left and right hands to avoid a learning effect, and that anxiety is the most common cause of errors. Observe for motor perseveration.
- Abstract thinking and conceptualization: proverbs (e.g. 'People in glass houses shouldn't throw stones'); similarities and differences (e.g. child and dwarf).
- Cognitive estimates test (e.g. largest object in a household room).
- Go–no–go tests: 'You tap once when I tap twice, you tap twice when I tap once.' Important to check the patient has understood the instruction.

Occipital lobe lesions

These can lead to simple or complex visual hallucinations, as well as difficulties with visual recognition. Severely, cortical blindness is seen.

Corpus callosal lesions

These can lead to callosal disconnection syndromes and severe and rapid intellectual deterioration.

Diencephalic and brainstem lesions

These can lead to Korsakoff-type amnesia (especially deep midline), rapidly progressive dementia with intellectual deterioration secondary to hydrocephalus, frontal-type syndrome (with better insight), hypersomnia, emotional lability, stupor, akinetic mutism, pseudobulbar palsy, and hypothalamic disorders.

The approach to the cognitive and neuropsychiatric assessment should, like all examinations, be interpreted in the context of the history and the overall state of the patient. If in doubt, think laterally and try an alternative test of the same function. Ask yourself if the findings make sense in terms of the presentation and differential, rather than seeing them as absolute findings. Performance on bedside tests is very dependent on factors such as expectations, language, and level of anxiety.

Further reading

Kopelman, M.D. (1994). Structured psychiatric interview: assessment of the cognitive state. *British Journal of Hospital Medicine*, 52, 277–81.
Hodges, J.R. (1994). *Cognitive Assessment for Clinicians*. Oxford University Press.

Neurological examination

A comprehensive neurological examination should be within the skill of every psychiatrist but it is useful to be able to perform a quick screening test as described here.

Note **handedness** by watching the patient write. Examine eye movements and visual fields. **Gait** (Table 5.2) is a good way of testing voluntary movement. Ask the patient to walk placing one foot in front of the other, as though on a tightrope (**tandem gait test**). **Sitting** or other resting posture allows observation of involuntary movements.

Motor function can further be assessed by asking the patient to extend their arms, rapidly move the fingers (as though playing the piano), and then to hold the arms outstretched (watch for drift).

Note any abnormal movements and describe them (Table 5.3).

Reflexes can be quickly tested with a tendon hammer once the patient is sitting or recumbent. Hyper-reflexic tendon jerks are most commonly due to anxiety. An up-going (positive) plantar or Babinski reflex indicates an upper motor neuron lesion.

Testing of **sensation** may be performed if the history indicates a deficit. Peripheral neuropathy is probably the most common positive finding and may be due to diabetes, alcohol, or lead poisoning.

Table 5.2 Assessing stance and gait

Deficit	Appearance	Confirmatory signs	Neuropsychiatric associations
Hemiplegic	Arm and hand flexed and internally rotated	Increased tone, brisk reflexes, upgoing plantar	Depression is common post-CVA (especially in anterior lesions?) Hemiplegias acquired in childhood may lead to preserved language function at the expense of visuospatial skills, regardless of lesion site
Parkinsonian	Stooped posture, reduced arm swing, bradykinesia, shuffling gait which improves with afferent input (e.g. walking with a friend)	'Lead-pipe' rigidity, 'pill-rolling' tremor which combine to give 'cogwheeling' Paucity of speech and facial expression	Drug-induced (where tremor uncommon) seen more than PD Personality change (obsessionality and hypochondriasis) said to characterize PD Dementia: 10–15% increasing with duration of disease Frontal-like syndrome (subcortical dementia) Depression common but unrelated to stage of disease; psychosis usually iatrogenic Note: impulse control disorders with dopaminergic agents
Cerebellar	Wide-based stance and gait, slurred speech	Dysmetria (past pointing), intention tremor, nystagmus	Possible current intoxication (alcohol, lithium, anticonvulsants) or chronic damage (e.g. MS; look for pale disks, pyramidal signs) or alcoholism
Akathisia	Motor restlessness, inability to sit or stand still	Subjective sense of inner distress and motor tension	Present in 20–30% of patients on neuroleptics; often overlooked

CVA, cerebrovascular accident; PD, Parkinson's disease; MS, multiple sclerosis.

Table 5.3 Assessing and describing abnormal movements

Deficit	Appearance	Confirmatory signs	Neuropsychiatric associations
Choreiform	Rapid irregular dance-like or jerky involuntary movements	Consider more detailed cognitive testing	Huntington's disease Accompanying medical condition (e.g. SLE, pregnancy, thyrotoxicosis) Drug-induced OCP, neuroleptics, phenytoin Basal ganglia vascular disease, neuroacanthocytosis,
Tic disorders	Repeated jerky movements, mimicking normal actions and under some voluntary control	Ask about suppressibility, and OCP	Common in children but reduce with age; usually affect periocular muscles, face, neck, and shoulders Gilles de la Tourette syndrome implies motor and vocal tics
Dystonic	Sustained muscular contractions cause repetitive twisting movements, or abnormal postures and bizarre gaits; may occur focally (e.g. writer's cramp, spasmodic torticollis	Recheck medication history: neuroleptics, antiemetics, SSRIs, and lithium have been implicated	Acute dystonia rapidly relieved by anticholinergics Tardive dystonia is difficult to treat and can be very disabling Rarer causes include Wilson's disease (look for associated basal ganglia and liver disease) and Huntington's disease

SLE, systemic lupus erythematosus; OCP, obsessive–compulsive phenomena; SSRI, selective serotonin reuptake inhibitor.

Specific scenarios

1. The patient with functional symptoms

In assessing a patient with suspected non-organic symptoms, you should be aware of the following:

- Many patients with functional disorders will have no other obvious psychopathology, so do not see the interview as merely a 'screening' for depression, anxiety, or other mental illness.
- Acknowledging the somatic symptoms is important, so invest some time in hearing these—if they are very many, however, it may help to 'make a list' and avoid a detailed history of each symptom.
- Try and get a good idea of the time course of the symptoms.
- Acknowledge the patient may feel puzzled, angry, or suspicious about being asked to see a psychiatrist.
- Avoid too rapid conclusions or diagnoses.
- May be useful to use analogies—for example, between 'hardware' and 'software' problems or 'blocks'.
- May be useful to consider if the patient has had the experience of being 'not believed' or 'fobbed off'—acknowledging these experiences can help engage the patient in a non-medical model of illness.
- Avoid overly simplistic observations but acknowledge that functional recovery *should* be possible in the absence of hard neurological damage.

2. The mute or inaccessible patient

Definitions

Mutism is the inability or unwillingness to speak, resulting in the absence or marked paucity of verbal output. It may be isolated or associated with other disturbances of behaviour, level of consciousness, affect, motor disturbance, or thought processes. There are organic and non-organic causes. **Stupor** constitutes preserved awareness with severe psychomotor inhibition. Mutism is invariably present in stupor. In general, these terms should not be used in isolation, but should be combined with a detailed description of the clinical features.

History

The history will need to be obtained from informants. How long has the patient been mute? Was the development sudden or gradual? Was there a stressful precipitant, or did the patient seem overly sad or happy in the prodrome? Is the mutism partial or complete? Is it specific to one situation (e.g. school)? Does any of the patient's behaviour seem odd or bizarre? How does the patient function in everyday life: eating, drinking, sleeping, continence, social activities, etc.? Is there a past history of psychiatric disorder, conversion disorder, or neurological or medical illness? What drugs have been prescribed/taken?

Examination

A general examination of physical state—temperature, pulse, blood pressure, and state of hydration (look at the tongue)—should be undertaken. The presence of mutism also demands a full neurological examination, beginning with an assessment of the level of consciousness. An impaired level of consciousness or the presence of focal neurological signs should lead to prompt referral to a physician or neurologist.

Specifically, check whether the patient can articulate (by making lip movements or whispering) or phonate (by humming or coughing). Take note of the eye movements. Is the patient watchful and/or making purposive movements implying awareness of surroundings? Are the eyes deviated to one side or another? (Non-organic states may be indicated by eyes deviating to alternate sides depending on the position of the head.) Does the patient with closed eyes resist opening? Is re-closure of the eyes slow and uniform, as occurs in the unconscious patient (and not usually possible to simulate), or is there resistance?

Is communication possible by other means (e.g. writing/signing)? Are there any attempts to speak? To what extent is comprehension affected? (Pure motor (Broca's) dysphasia is normally accompanied by frustrated attempts at communication and comprehension is relatively intact.)

Mental state

Note the state of mental arousal and motor activity. Is there associated motor retardation? What is indicated by facial expression? Does s/he appear elated, anxious, frightened, sad, or angry? Describe any grimaces, gestures, or mannerisms. Is there any evidence of attempts at communication, or does the patient seem unconcerned by his/her state (e.g. is there 'belle indifference')? Does s/he appear to be preoccupied, perhaps by hallucinations, ruminations, or paranoia? It may be appropriate to describe the mental state as inaccessible if the patient appears alert but you are unable to establish meaningful communication.

Differential diagnosis of mutism

Psychiatric disorders

- **Psychotic disorder**: mutism may occur as a response to a delusional system in schizophrenia or as part of the negative symptoms in association with reduced drive. Strong experiences of passivity may result in a stupor.
- **Affective disorder**: mutism in depression may result in psychomotor retardation or nihilism, whereas in mania it may occur as part of a manic stupor.
- **Elective mutism**: this is most often seen in children, where there is emotionally determined selectivity in speaking; it is associated with social anxiety, withdrawal, or sensitivity.
- **Pervasive developmental disorders**: the use of language is delayed and often idiosyncratic, although mutism is rare. It is accompanied by impairments in social interaction and a restricted range of interests.
- **Obsessional slowness**: this may be accompanied by severely restricted speech output.
- **Somatoform/dissociative disorder**: in psychogenic dysphonia, the ability to phonate may help in differentiating it from an organic condition. Post-traumatic stress disorder may also be accompanied by mutism.
- **Factitious disorder**: this is rare, but may occur in situations where divulgence of information may be detrimental (e.g. with a pending court case).

Neurological disorders

- **Lesions** of cortex (e.g. frontal, speech areas), brainstem (e.g. akinetic mutism: coma vigil, 'locked in syndrome'), basal ganglia (e.g. Parkinson's disease, Wilson's disease).
- **Infective**: herpes encephalitis, HIV-related disease.
- **Drugs**: neuroleptics (may cause dystonic reactions involving tongue and jaw muscles, as well as torticollis, laryngeal spasm, and oculogyric crises), lithium, sedatives, antiepileptics.
- **Seizure-related**: during or after complex partial seizures, absence attacks, partial status.
- **Deafness**: may give rise to speech delay in children and impaired production of speech.

Investigations

Investigations should include haematology, biochemistry (including blood sugar), toxin/drug/infective screen, endocrine screen, chest radiography, EEG (which may indicate localized epileptiform activity or the generalized slowing of encephalopathies, although its absence does not necessarily exclude seizures), and brain imaging with CT or MRI.

Initial treatment

Once serious neurological disorder has been excluded, a period of observation is often valuable, although the presence of severe psychomotor retardation in depressive disorder or manic stupor may require urgent treatment and electroconvulsive therapy (ECT) should be considered. Treatment of dystonic reactions should be initiated rapidly, as they are frightening and painful for patients. Intravenous or intramuscular procyclidine or benztropine is effective.

3. The catatonic patient

Definition

Catatonia is a term that causes confusion because of its historical association with a particular presentation of schizophrenia. It is a non-specific syndrome that occurs in a variety of organic states as well as in psychotic, affective, and somatoform psychiatric disorders and in association with autism. Catatonia is characterized by abnormal motor behaviours, with periods of hyper- and hypoactivity. Mutism and stupor are common, and it is often associated with features such as posturing, waxy flexibility, negativism, impulsiveness, stereotypies, mannerisms, command automatisms, echopraxia, or echolalia.

History

The ability of the catatonic patient to give a history may be preserved, and history-taking should then proceed along normal lines. More commonly, however, communication is impaired, and assessment must be undertaken as for the mute patient, questioning relevant informants. If communication is possible, the patient should be asked about any meaning attached to the postures adopted, which may lead to the uncovering of a delusional system, the degree to which the patient is distressed by the motor symptoms (it is important to distinguish from the mental and physical agitation of neuroleptic-induced akathisia), and whether passive movement is painful (which is often the case in waxy flexibility). Also ask about previous episodes of catatonia, as well as past psychiatric history.

Examination

As with mutism, the presence of catatonia demands full physical examination. Patients may shift rapidly into a period of catatonic overactivity, which could render people close by in physical danger; therefore, vigilance should be retained during examination. The catatonic patient is at risk of dehydration, rhabdomyolysis, sepsis, venous thrombosis, and pressure sores, and examination should pay particular attention to these factors as well as excluding the organic causes of catatonia. The following phenomena should be elicited where possible:

- automatic obedience: a robot-like response to any instruction, however silly
- negativism: a similarly stereotyped response, but the opposite of what was requested
- waxy flexibility: the patient's limbs can be moved slowly into a new posture passively, but return gradually to the previously sustained posture
- 'psychological pillow': on lying down, the patient's head remains held a few inches above the bed
- ambitendence: the patient begins to make a movement, but before completing it begins to make the opposite movement
- echolalia: the patient repeats the examiner's words or phrases
- echopraxia: the patient repeats any movements made by the examiner
- mannerisms: repetitive goal-directed behaviour
- stereotypies: repetitive non-goal-directed behaviours.

Sometimes in the mute, stuporose, or catatonic patient, it is not possible to access the mental state. In these cases, it may be important to keep an open mind as to organic or non-organic aetiologies. Benzodiazepines, often in high doses, may relieve the symptoms of catatonia and facilitate access to the patient's mental state.

Differential diagnosis

Psychiatric disorders

- **Affective disorder**: depression is probably the most common psychiatric cause of catatonia and is considerably more common than mania. It often develops slowly; therefore, the history may be particularly informative.
- **Schizophrenic disorder**: 'catatonic schizophrenia' is relatively rarely diagnosed, although catatonic motor disorders (i.e. a part of the catatonic syndrome) are commonly seen in all subgroups of schizophrenia. Catatonia is a relatively common presentation of puerperal psychosis.
- **Obsessional slowness**: catatonic features may be due to severe obsessive–compulsive disorder. Access to the typical mental state (with ruminations and obsessions) may be available with observation or from the informant's history.

- **Somatoform/dissociative**: this is rare and requires both the absence of physical and functional psychiatric aetiology, as well as positive evidence of psychogenic causation.

Neurological disorders
- **Lesions** of cortex (frontal and temporal lobes), brainstem, basal ganglia, limbic system, or diencephalon (e.g. tumour, cerebral thrombosis or haemorrhage, head injury, infection including encephalitis lethargica and syphilis).
- **Drugs**: neuroleptics (neuroleptic malignant syndrome—catatonia with rigidity and temperature/autonomic instability), lithium, morphine derivatives.
- **Toxins**: carbon monoxide poisoning, alcohol damage, ecstasy, alcohol.
- **Seizure-related**: simple partial or complex partial seizures.
- **Systemic**: renal or hepatic failure, endocrine disorders, connective tissue disorders (particularly cerebral systemic lupus erythematosus).
- **Other**: acute intermittent or coproporphyria, vitamin deficiency.

In addition, there are a proportion of patients who present with recurrent catatonia in whom no psychiatric or neurological disorder can be found. This subgroup seems to be familial, and spontaneous recovery is the general rule.

Investigations
Advice is similar to that already given for the mute or stuporose patient. In the case of diagnostic difficulty, abreaction (usually with benzodiazepine) may reverse the catatonia of the functional psychoses for a short time, allowing the emergence of 'hidden' psychopathology. The response to a single session of ECT may also be useful diagnostically.

Initial treatment
Supportive treatment, including fluid and electrolyte replacement, antibiotics, and anticoagulation should be initiated where indicated. Once treatable neurological causes have been excluded, consideration should be given to the early or even emergency use of ECT, as patients are at risk of a number of physical complications. Benzodiazepines, intravenously and then orally, have been shown to be of value acutely. Neuroleptics may be effective in the presence of psychosis.

Neuroleptic malignant syndrome should be considered a medical emergency, and advice should be sought urgently. Initial treatment is discontinuation of the neuroleptic, supportive treatment of autonomic and temperature regulation failure, and treatment with dantrolene, benzodiazepines, and dopamine agonists (see 'Neuroleptic malignant syndrome', p. 134).

The formulation, the summary, and progress notes

A **summary** is a descriptive account of collected data; it is objective and impartial. In contrast, a **formulation** is a clinical opinion, weighing up the pros and cons of conflicting evidence, which leads to a diagnostic choice and a recommended management plan for an individual patient. An opinion inevitably implies a subjective viewpoint, or value judgement, by virtue of assigning relative importance to each piece of evidence; in doing so, both theoretical bias and past personal experiences invariably come into play. No matter how accurate, a formulation is inextricably bound up with subjective judgements and decisions. When assessing the same patient, two experts may produce two similar summaries, but two different formulations. This is the fundamental difference: a *summary* is descriptive, whereas a *formulation* is analytical and evaluative. Therefore, a summary calls for the qualities of thoroughness, restraint, and objectivity, whereas a formulation demands the composite skill of methodical thinking, incisive and imaginative analysis, and intelligent presentation.

Formulating a case with clarity and precision is probably the most testing yet most challenging and crucial part of a psychiatric assessment. The skill of writing a good formulation depends upon the ability to differentiate the merely incidental and circumstantial biographical details from the salient and discriminatory features forming the cornerstone of a clinical diagnosis. Certain features are discriminatory because they support one diagnosis as the more likely candidate and discount another diagnosis as less likely. Formulation also aims to pick out the most relevant causative factors for the individual patient (biological, psychological, or social)—identification of which drives a management plan likely to help.

The formulation

A diagnosis involves a **nomothetic** (literally 'law-giving') process. This means that all cases included within the identified category have one or more properties in common thereby making the category general. In contrast, the formulation is an **idiographic** process (literally 'picture of the individual'). This means that it includes the unique characteristics of each patient's case, needed for the process of management. Therefore, while nomothetic processes are the only way we can advance knowledge about diseases, we use idiographic methods to understand and study the individual.

The format of the formulation
The formulation follows a logical sequence.

Demographic data
Begin with the patient's name, age, occupation, and marital status.

Descriptive formulation
Describe the nature of onset (e.g. acute or insidious), the total duration of the present illness, and the course (e.g. cyclic or deteriorating). Then list the main phenomena (i.e. symptoms and signs) characterizing the disorder. As you become more experienced, you should try to be selective by featuring the phenomena that are most important because of either their greater diagnostic specificity or their predominance in severity or duration. Avoid long lists of minor or transient symptoms and negative findings, but include

those that help to exclude other possible diagnoses. These basic data are chiefly derived from the history of the present illness, the mental state, and physical examinations, and are used to determine the syndrome diagnosis in the next section. Note that this is not usually the place to bring in other aspects of the history; that comes later. If we know the diagnosis of a previous episode of mental illness, this should also be taken into account, but remember that the present disorder may not be connected and the diagnosis may be different.

Differential diagnosis

List, in order of probability, all disorders that you will wish to investigate. These will usually be syndrome diagnoses based on the descriptive formulation just described. Give the evidence for and against each diagnosis that you consider. Include any current physical illness that may account for some or all of the phenomena. A common error is to include, for example, thyroid function studies in the investigations without including thyroid disease in the differential diagnosis. If you think that a condition is worth investigating, then you are obviously including it in your differential diagnosis; if it is not worth mentioning, then do not bother to investigate it.

Remember that you will frequently need to consider supplementary diagnoses in addition to the primary diagnosis; for example, alcohol dependence in a patient presenting with delirium, or a personality disorder in a patient with an anxiety state.

Aetiology

The various factors that have contributed should be evident mainly from the family and personal histories, the history of previous illness, and the premorbid personality. It may be helpful to order aetiological factors by making reference to the biopsychosocial model of illness. This suggests that you organize the aetiological factors relevant to an individual presentation according to biological, psychological, and social factors, subdividing each domain into predisposing, precipitating, and perpetuating factors. Try to answer two questions: Why has this patient developed this particular disorder? Why has the disorder developed at this particular time?

Investigations

List all investigations that are required to support your preferred diagnosis and to rule out the alternatives, and also any that you think are necessary to improve your understanding of the aetiology. Give reasons for investigations if they are not self-evident. Remember that the thorough investigation of an illness requires effective enquiry into biological, psychological, and social domains; be willing to include psychological investigations as well as relevant social enquiry.

Treatment

Outline the treatment plan that you wish to follow. This should stem logically from your discussion of the aetiology as well as from the diagnosis.

Prognosis

Describe the expected outcome of management of this illness episode, with regard to both the symptoms and subsequent function (e.g. self-care and return to the community). Consider the risk of subsequent relapse.

The summary

This is an important document and should be drawn up with care. Its purpose is to provide a concise description of all the important aspects of the case to enable others who are unfamiliar with the patient to grasp the essential features of the problem without needing to search elsewhere for further information.

The first part should be completed within a week of admission and be arranged under the following headings:

- reason for referral and referrer
- family history
- personal history
  - childhood
  - occupations
  - marriage/partnership and children
  - premorbid personality
  - physical illness
  - previous mental illness
- medication and treatment history
- physical examination
- mental state.

The summary of the psychiatric examination should cover all important aspects of the mental state and be drawn up under whichever of the subheadings in the main schema are necessary to achieve this. The six subheadings of personal history just listed should always be included, and others from the main schema introduced as appropriate.

The second part should be completed within a week of discharge and be laid out under the following headings:

- Investigations
- Treatment and progress
  - Include details of medication prescribed and response; also note any significant side effects or reasons for changing medication. Document any other therapeutic strategies introduced. It is also helpful to record any significant episodes during the admission.
- Final diagnosis (or diagnoses) together with the ICD-10 diagnostic code number
- Prognosis
  - Make a predictive statement related to symptoms and social adaptation, rather than terms like guarded, good, or poor.
- Condition on discharge
- Discharge medication
- Follow up arrangements and care plan

The completed summary should be short enough to occupy about two sides of A4 paper. A summary is necessarily a compromise between the need to document all the significant aspects of an admission and economy. The summary of a re-admission should include the full range of categories listed here, unless the last admission was very recent and it has been established that no significant change has occurred in the family history and personal history in the interim.

References to highly confidential matters (criminal acts, sexual revelations, etc.) should be included only if their omission would produce serious distortion of the overall picture. Often it will be preferable to include only a limited reference followed by 'see notes' in parentheses. The summary should identify which professional workers are to be responsible for different aspects of the patient's care in the future.

Progress notes

Regular progress notes, or event notes, *signed and dated*, are a vital part of every case record. They should describe the treatment that the patient is receiving (with dates of starting and finishing, and dosages of all drugs), significant changes in mental state, and any important events involving the patient. They should also record the opinions expressed by consultants at ward rounds and case conferences. In particular, you should document the reasons supporting significant changes in management. Although these notes must be detailed enough to convey an accurate picture of the patient's treatment and his/her response to it, they should not normally contain lengthy verbatim accounts of conversations between patient and doctor. Notes that are excessively long are never read.

Handover notes

A handover note should be written whenever the patient is transferred from the care of one junior doctor to another, summarizing the salient features and outlining future plans. This is particularly important in the case of outpatients for whom there is no formal summary or formulation.

Special interview situations

The patient who demands proof that you care

Some socially isolated people rely on their doctors and other professionals for a large part of their social contact. Some accept the limitations and boundaries of the professional relationship and operate within it by generating the kinds of problems they know that you will deal with: new or troublesome side effects or non-specific somatic complaints, for example. A small number end up making escalating demands on the clinician based on the assertion that you really do not care and it is only a professional relationship to you.

In order to demonstrate that you do care, you may find yourself putting them at the end of an outpatient clinic so that you can spend longer with them than with other patients. Then you may find that everyone else has gone home by the time you finish their consultation. As you recognize the person's desperate state, you may give them your direct number and encourage him or her to telephone you between appointments. Then, as it becomes clear that once-weekly visits to the clinic are insufficient, you find yourself offering extra appointments outside of working hours. By this time, you have a 'special patient', although often none of your tokens of care are having the desired effect. Far from the patient becoming happier and more able to face life independently, you are now indispensable to this special patient's survival. Indeed, suicide threats and gestures may appear to ensure that you remain centrally involved to their care. Frightened, vulnerable behaviour may elicit an impulse to comfort the patient—holding hands, even an arm round the shoulder. However, you need to recognize and resist this temptation: you are allowing yourself to be drawn into a compromising situation.

It is not that such people are not unwell, and have not suffered significant deprivation. It is more that you will not be able to prove that you care enough. The danger for you is that a central motivation in becoming a doctor—the relief of suffering and the wish to heal—is being distorted and your professional integrity is under threat. Sexual contact between doctor and patient is not uncommon, and may be the result of a series of short steps, that can start as outlined here. It is an unequivocal breach of professional ethics.

The cardinal rule in caring for patients who demand proof, by whatever means, that you care, is not to become isolated with them. The first step is to ensure that you are well supervised and supported by peers and senior colleagues, and the second is to arrive at a care plan that involves the multidisciplinary team. Psychodynamic supervision of such cases is a helpful but increasingly scarce resource to optimize the care and protect those involved.

The patient who solicits erotic involvement

From time to time a patient may develop an erotic attachment to their doctor and declare or act on it. Sometimes this can be managed by simply explaining that it is impossible for you to continue as their doctor if you are treated as a potential lover. Indeed, this may be the unconscious motivation of the patient's attraction, so that one could pose the question: 'What is it about my being your doctor that you wish to avoid?'. Assessment of the underlying disturbance is essential, as such declarations may (among others) be the expression of extreme social isolation, the manifestation of a personality disorder, or the presentation of a potentially complex and even dangerous psychotic disorder. Whatever the disturbance, if the patient persists importunately there is no alternative but to transfer care to a colleague, explaining that further contact between you and the patient will cease. Further harassment and stalking are matters for your colleague, and possibly a forensic psychiatrist and the police.

When such cases arise it is important to examine one's own presentation and behaviour to ensure that one is not unconsciously signalling availability or even behaving seductively towards the patient. Again, good-quality and regular supervision of such cases from a senior colleague and possibly a psychotherapist is what is needed to support you. Supervision is also valuable as you tread the delicate balance between not giving the patient any encouragement and not inflicting unnecessary humiliation.

The patient who brings gifts

In psychiatry, one probably expects expressions of gratitude less often than in some specialities. Nevertheless, patients do bring gifts from time to time. There may be no problem with a parting gift at the end of a course of treatment, when it is often appropriate to accept it graciously, unless it is cash. Gifts presented during the course of treatment are more likely to be complicated and may contain another message. Find a way of addressing this without being churlish. For example, work the patient has done in the context of treatment (pottery in occupational therapy, a poem, or a painting) may be important signs of competence and recovery; they may also be a concrete token of the patient's wish to remain in your mind and be part of your non-professional life. This is better put into words than left unspoken, and acceptance of the gift may be appropriate when the air has been cleared.

More extravagant and inappropriate gifts might suggest that the patient has privately elevated you, to be placated and propitiated, and perhaps expects untold benefits in return one day. This is a more direct attack on the professional relationship and needs to be addressed: 'I really cannot accept such an expensive gift; I wonder if you fear I will not take you seriously if you come empty-handed', or some variation on this.

The patient who is disinhibited

At its most harmless, disinhibition might take the form of personal remarks, tactless jokes, or personal questions. Do not rise to personal remarks or laugh at tactless jokes, and fend off intrusive personal questions. In general, respond in a muted, subdued, professional manner, avoiding perpetuating the inappropriate tone.

More difficult to deal with is the patient who enters your personal space to touch or stroke you. Depending on the patient's mental state, and with the milder forms of intrusion, you might try distraction; for example, 'You were telling me about the voices that you hear'. More overt intrusion is less easily dealt with, and you may have to withdraw and try again later, or return with a chaperone. It is especially important to do this if examining a sexually disinhibited patient of either gender. Physical aggression calls for back-up, and you should always have access to a call button.

The patient who refuses to leave

Rise at the end of the consultation to signal clearly that the session is over. Say, 'I am sorry, I am going to have to ask you to leave'. You can appeal to the person's better nature: 'If you don't go now I will be keeping others waiting' (this of course may be the reason that the patient will not leave). Finally, say 'I am going to call for someone to help you out of my room' and telephone for help. This is probably preferable to any attempt to coax or manhandle the patient alone.

The patient out of hours

Be prepared and expect the unexpected. Many awkward situations arise because the doctor has been only half awake to the fact that people, at least from time to time, do not behave reasonably. Do not be overconfident or complacent.

If you are called out of hours to see a patient whom you do not know, on a ward or in A&E, in so far as it is possible, prepare. Inform yourself about him/her before the interview. Read the medical and nursing notes, especially the admission summary, formulations, care plans, and reports of ward-round decisions. Look at the risk assessment and the elements of the care plans. Ask to be updated on the most recent events and presentation by the senior nurse on duty and speak to any accompanying carer. Where possible, ask a member of the nursing team to be with you while you interview the patient for the first time, and never conduct a physical examination alone. If you do decide to interview the patient on your own, first of all be clear about how to call for help.

Make sure that the nurses know where you are and develop a contingency plan. Position yourself within reach of the telephone and know the number to call for help. Talk to the nurse in charge and make sure that there is somebody within earshot who knows to respond quickly if there are signs of agitation. If there is a 'panic button', know where it is and keep it within reach. It is safer to position the patient away from the door, leaving your path out uncluttered. If the patient produces a weapon, terminate the interview as quickly as you can by explaining to the patient that it is impossible for you to help someone who is armed, but that the consultation can be resumed once the weapon has been handed over for safe keeping. Leave as soon as you have said this, if the patient will allow you to do so; offer to fetch a cup of tea or coffee to allow the opportunity to think about what you have said. If the patient will not allow you to leave, stay calm and chat to him/her about neutral matters; if you can press the panic button without risk, do so.

The patient who demands drugs

Often the story given is one of a lost prescription or of sudden motivation to stop illicit drug use. There are no rules about how to deal with this situation but the following points may help.

- Take a good history of exactly which drugs and how much the patient is consuming. Is there a history of dependence? Are there objective features of withdrawal?
- If s/he claims to have lost a prescription, who was it prescribed by? Can you check with them? Where is it being dispensed? When was it last dispensed? Do they collect only or is their consumption supervised? Pharmacists keep good records and will often be open late.
- Do not prescribe unless you feel confident that you are doing so safely. Be aware of the maximum safe doses. Be aware of the need to monitor physical parameters.
- Remember that opiate withdrawal is not physically dangerous but benzodiazepine withdrawal and alcohol withdrawal can be.
- The patient has probably been using illicit drugs for a long time. S/he can continue for another day or two until an appropriate referral is made.
- Try to consult a specialist.

The patient who threatens violence

Even the most skilful clinician will occasionally be faced with a patient whose behaviour escalates to the point that physical aggression and violence seem imminent (but see Chapter 1, 'The A&E setting', p. 9). Usually, this arises when some real or perceived threat to his/her physical or psychological integrity has made the patient either very frightened or very angry—essentially, that things are getting out of his/her control. Particularly high-risk situations include interviewing patients whose persecutory delusional beliefs are that harm is imminent, or telling a patient of a clinical decision to detain or treat him/her against his/her will. Patients who are disinhibited by drugs or alcohol or their mental state are especially prone to sudden impulsive aggression.

A lot can be done to defuse a situation before violence erupts, and not just for your own benefit—the staff and security will avoid the risks of having to come to your aid, and the patient will escape adverse labelling and, possibly, even a criminal charge. Anticipate your interview with an unknown, possibly disturbed patient by doing the following.

- Read the records for information about the patient's likely mental state and any previous history of violence and substance misuse, and the circumstances.
- Read the old risk assessments, paying particular attention to early warning signs.
- Ask the nursing staff and carers about his/her current presentation and concerns, and whether they think s/he is intoxicated. Junior nursing staff will often defer to you on the question as to whether the patient appears safe to interview alone (even if you know far less about him/her than they do) unless you make it clear that you value their views.
- Arrange to use an interview room that can be easily observed by staff who know where you are, or who are prepared to wait outside if necessary. Has the patient been searched? Ideally, the room should have an alarm button that is close to hand and the door should be easily opened from the inside. Think about safe seating arrangements and ensure that you have an unobstructed route to the door.
- Equally, the room should also allow for a degree of privacy and be quiet.

The interview itself should be conducted in a measured, polite, and professional manner; not only will this promote a psychological distance between you and the patient, which discourages violence, but by treating him/her appropriately, you will increase his/her self-esteem. Do not invade his/her personal space, touch him/her, tower over, stare, or sit behind a large desk; rather, make an effort to build a rapport. Tell the patient who you are and that you want to do your best to help. Take time to listen to his/her concerns, and if they are delusional, acknowledge his/her fear, distress, or anger rather than arguing about their veracity.

It often helps to tell the patient that s/he is frightening people, as s/he may genuinely be unaware of this.

These techniques will fail with some patients, especially if they are intoxicated, have very fixed beliefs, or are very aroused. If your intuition tells you that all is not well, listen to it. If you are clearly getting nowhere in an interview, do not increase the patient's frustration by prolonging the interview unnecessarily. Typically, the matter can only be resolved by telling the patient that you want him/her to do something, such as stay in hospital, take medication, or go into the seclusion room. By now, you will know that this is going to be provocative, and if you are alone with him/her it will be best to leave the room and fetch help; if necessary, tell the patient that you are going to consult a senior colleague. Confronting such a patient with medication should only be done with a suitably trained and staffed team in the room with you, and with the medication prepared and ready to be administered. Ensure that suitable physical health monitoring can be implemented as well.

The assessment of violence risk

The general approach to the problem of violence has shifted; the central focus is now the assessment of the risk of violence that s/he poses in a particular situation under specific circumstances, rather than whether or not they are dangerous. This paradigm shift has facilitated clearer and more structured thinking about the factors that contribute to patients' potential violent behaviour. This process highlights the importance of risk factors, and the quality of the information on which our decisions are based, and their underlying supporting evidence.

Theoretical framework

Recognize that some level of risk is present

Just as the psychiatrist must now consider the risk of suicide, so thinking about whether a patient may pose a risk of harm to others has become routine. As with suicide, sometimes the risk of violence is unmistakable. However, on many occasions it will be much less so. While apparently obvious, it needs to be stressed that recognizing that the risk exists is the essential first step in the assessment process. Actuarial data help estimate the probability of violence in an individual by considering their membership of a group. This demonstrates the limits to predicting violence in an individual due to low base rates, even in acutely ill groups. Violence risk most clearly exists in patient groups where there is a history of violence.

A process for risk assessment

Having become aware that there is a risk, the psychiatrist should aim to be able to define for that patient:
- the **nature** of the risk, with some sort of estimate of the likely **seriousness** of the potential harm
- an estimate of the **probability** that the risk will materialize (this should be based on actuarial data where available)
- an estimate of the **imminence** that the risk will become reality.

Formulate a plan of management to reduce risk(s)

Having answered these questions, the psychiatrist should then aim to develop a risk management plan. The plan will utilize and act on the information about the presence and relevance of factors identified in the risk assessment, and aim to address or minimize each of them. The plan should address the factors that have been identified to contribute to the risk. It is always important to remember the importance of an explicit time-scale. Risk assessment becomes less accurate the further into the future it stretches; re-assessment of the patient's risk and re-evaluation of the risk management plan's performance are important aspects.

Practical risk assessment

The structure and nature of risk assessments will necessarily vary according to the case and the circumstances. Those completed in the context of a decision to transfer from high to medium security will differ from those carried out in A&E overnight. It is not only a question of the differing resources and information available. The purposes of the assessments, the relative urgency of the decisions that need to be taken, and the period for which such decisions can be considered to remain accurate are all completely different.

The practical process of risk assessment can be thought of in three stages: gathering and reviewing all the **documentary information** from all relevant sources; **examining the patient and interviewing informants**; and **asking yourself questions** concerning the patient, the circumstances, and the potential victims. From the documentation and interviews, the psychiatrist should aim to gain as complete a picture as is feasible of the possible unwanted behaviour and its antecedents. In forensic circles this is called 'scenario planning' and is linked to the concept of risk formulation.

Factors to include

The index incident
Most obviously, risk assessment is needed for patients who have already been or have threatened violence. In such cases, it is important to record a detailed account of the index incident and its antecedents. The patient may be able to provide an initial picture which may, but may not, minimize the violence. An independent perspective from a third party is of great value; for example, from nurses or witness statements, depending on the circumstances of the incident. In addition to providing detail of the violent incident, witness statements often give a sharp narrative of the real impact of the behaviour—an impact which is often lost as the story is repeated and adulterated through successive accounts.

Analysing such accounts of the index behaviour should be targeted at developing an understanding of the patient's prevailing mental state at that time and the factors (e.g. psychosis, emotional state, alcohol or drug use) that might have contributed to it, both in the medium and short term. Were they angry, afraid, or lacking an emotional response? Were his/her actions planned (even if psychotically motivated), impulsive, or a response to a new precipitant? Did they use a weapon?

The immediate and medium-term antecedents and destabilizers
The immediate antecedents of the index violence should be explored from several angles to gain an understanding of the precipitating factors. The patient may have suffered or be threatened by the loss of someone important. S/he may have experienced rejection or loss of face. His/her accommodation or financial security might have been at risk. S/he may have refused medication or increased his/her misuse of drugs or alcohol. Evidence of relapse may be evident without obvious cause. A pattern of change may be evident in the patient's life, culminating in the index offence. S/he may have become increasingly socially isolated and withdrawn, or moved away from home. Social restlessness or disengagement can be an ominous sign in the histories of particular psychotic perpetrators of violence.

Thought should be given as to how the patient's situation contributed to the index behaviour. Who was s/he in contact with? Was the behaviour of friends or family a factor, for example by encouraging drug or alcohol use or by discouraging compliance with supervision or treatment? Did the pattern of the patient's daily activities make the index behaviour more likely? Was the patient's accommodation appropriate?

The question of how or why the patient's victim was involved should be considered. Was the victim a stranger, an acquaintance, or a family member?

History from the patient

A comprehensive psychiatric history is an essential part of all risk assessments, with additional attention to certain specific domains.

1. A review of **previous violent behaviour** should be completed. All behaviour that brought the patient into contact with the police should be ascertained, with the outcome recorded in terms of conviction and sentence. Violent and criminal behaviour that did not come to police attention should also be recorded from as early as possible in the individual's life. Both inpatient and 'domestic' violence should not be neglected. Patterns, for example escalation in seriousness or decline in frequency, should be noted.

2. The patient's **exposure to violence**, both as victim and witness, should be noted. While the mechanism is poorly understood, victims of abuse are at increased risk of becoming perpetrators.

3. The patient's **psychiatric history** should be reconstructed with attention to such factors as mode of presentation, diagnosis, type of follow up and engagement with community supervision, nature of admission to hospital (e.g. voluntary or detained) and precipitating circumstances, the quality of treatment response, and the various facets of insight including both their illness and their risk, concordance and engagement with treatment and supervision, and their ability to seek effective help or support, or act on an illness and risk management plan. The success of community management or the reasons for its failure are of particular importance when decisions around admission and discharge are required. It may become clear that there is a constant relationship between psychiatric illness and violence and aggression, or that there is no relationship at all.

4. **Alcohol and drug misuse** must be assessed in detail due to their destabilizing and disinhibiting effects. Particular attention should be paid to the relationship between drug use and psychiatric illness, between drug use and treatment and supervision engagement, and between drug use and violence and aggression. These relationships are often complex; for example, violence when intoxicated may precede any mental illness, drug use may exacerbate pre-existing symptoms of mental illness associated with violence or increase impulsivity, drug use can be an attempt by the patient to 'treat' his/her symptoms, or criminal activity can be an attempt to finance a drug habit.

5. The **psychosexual and relationship history** should be explored. Childhood experience of physical or sexual abuse increases the chances that the adult will become a perpetrator. A pattern of short, unsuccessful intimate relationships, or an absolute lack of such, potentially indicates an inability to maintain quality adult relationships, which are considered to be stabilizing factors. Some understanding of the patient's attitudes to the opposite sex and sexual fantasies should be sought. Sexual psychopathology, including dysfunction or abnormal

sexual preference, should be noted, especially if the latter has been acted upon. Partners are relatively frequently the victims of violence associated with mental disorder.

Mental state

Just as a potentially suicidal patient should be asked about self-harm, so a potentially violent patient should be questioned explicitly about his/her thoughts, intentions, plans, and actions. S/he should be asked about specific victims, especially if threats have been made.

Although the evidence from studies at the group level is inconsistent, at the individual level, symptoms that may be particularly associated with violence in psychosis are delusions of persecution and of passivity. Acting on delusions is more likely if the delusions are associated with fear, suspicion, or anger. Threats made by the patient must be taken seriously, as should violent fantasies. This applies as much to patients manifesting profound depression who suggest that their families would be better off dead as to threats to kill. Hallucinations need to be explored, especially looking for demeaning or threatening content as well as explicit commands, and the patient's understanding of them.

The patient's perception of their illness should be assessed in terms of his/her acceptance that s/he is ill, their agreement to take medication and to submit for supervision and monitoring, and his/her understanding of the true nature of their experiences and the risks it might engender.

An exploration of the patient's inner world is as important as the clarification of external circumstances. The personal meaning to the patient of precipitating factors and the resultant violence is as important as the actual event. This is similar to finding out whether someone who took an overdose of what might seem a trivial amount actually thought it was potentially lethal. It is not necessarily the action or its result, but the intention that is important. Complete denial of violence or denial of personal responsibility for it is potentially ominous, as is lack of remorse. The patient's attitude to treatment, supervision, and monitoring should be noted.

Relevant features of the patient's personality should be assessed. Personality strengths such as the ability to make friends, work, or cope with adversity may reduce risk. Deviousness or deceptiveness increases uncertainty and risk.

Risk assessment: synthesis

The aim of violence risk assessment is violence prevention. This, if done well, will have beneficial effects not just for the general public, but for patients, their families, and health care professionals too. Defining the nature and seriousness of the potential violence, the probability that it will occur, and its imminence requires making sense of often considerable amounts of information.

Risk assessment and risk management

To reiterate, the purpose of violence risk assessment is violence prevention by designing and implementing an appropriate risk management plan.

An effective plan will take and act on those aspects of the patient's situation and mental state identified from the assessment that require changing, and can be changed. It will also recognize and take account of those important influences on behaviour which are not susceptible to intervention.

Risk management plans should be monitored, to see what works and what does not. Long-term risk management involves a continuous process of risk assessment and re-evaluation, which might also confirm risk reduction or indicate where interventions have been unsuccessful. In other words, patient management is continuously subject to **monitoring and re-evaluation**.

The multidisciplinary team should determine the strategies and tactics for the management of patients who pose significant risk, especially for those team members who will have specific roles in management. Success depends on the effective functioning of the team and on the **clear apportioning of responsibilities** within the team. Poor communication both within the team and between the team and other agencies involved has repeatedly been held responsible for failures of management and the tragedies that have ensued.

Effective risk management involves breaking down a single large process into a series of smaller steps.

Plans should be made to address the relevant factors that were identified in the risk assessment. These interventions should be written into the risk management plan, so that someone coming to the case can see what is needed. The basic elements of a good risk management plan should include:

- Monitoring—what is the best way to monitor the patient's risk and pick up on a change in factors that might indicate that risk is changing? Under what circumstances should a reassessment be triggered?
- Treatments—what treatment, support, or rehabilitation strategies will you deliver to address the deficits or needs indentified in the risk assessment? What are the priorities? Which of these can and need to be targeted first? Which can wait?
- Supervision—what surveillance strategies should be implemented? What restrictions should be imposed?
- Victim safety planning—what steps can be taken to enhance the safety of the most likely potential victims?

All plans should include a provision for performance monitoring so that both successful and failed interventions can be noted and adjusted. Appropriate responses, and contingency plans in the event of a failure, should be clearly spelt out. It is obvious that risk management plans must take account of what resources are available to the managing team. It should also be obvious that if the plans are not working, due to insufficient resources, that the managing team have a responsibility to draw attention to this. Referral to a better resourced or more specialized team may be an option.

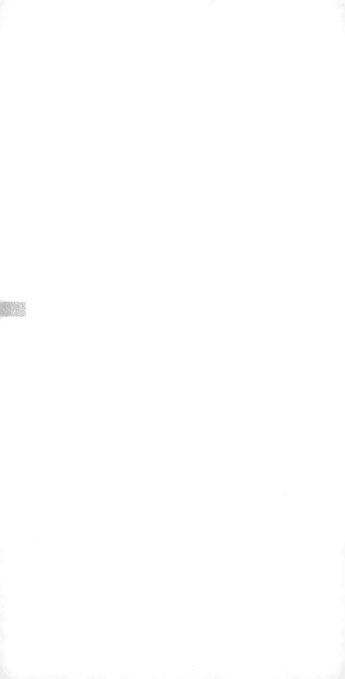

Special problems

Suicide and self-harm

How common is suicide?

Suicidal and self-harm behaviour is a significant public health problem. The annual rate of completed suicide in the UK is around 10 per 100,000, accounting for 1 per cent of all deaths. Self-harm presentations account for approximately 1 per cent of all Emergency Department presentations in the UK. Around 1 per cent of these presentations will die by suicide within a year, with risk highest in the first 6 months. It is important to note that not all self-harm behaviour has suicide as its intended outcome—there is often a complex mix of motivations. Appropriate assessment and management of the act itself, together with a strategy for prevention of repetition and suicide, is an essential skill for a psychiatrist.

Useful definitions

The concept 'suicidal behaviour' involves a continuum of behaviours ranging from suicidal thoughts to successful suicide. Full consensus on terminology has not yet been reached. The following definitions, based on ICD-10, will be used in this book:

- **Suicide:** a wilful self-inflicted act, which results in death.
- **Parasuicide:** a rather dated but still prevalent term relating to a non-fatal act in which an individual intentionally causes self-injury or ingests a substance in excess of any prescribed or generally recognized therapeutic dose. The term **suicide attempt** is often used in referring to cases of parasuicide involving intention to die.
- **Self-harm:** also previously labelled Deliberate Self-Harm (DSH) is an intentional non-fatal act committed in the knowledge that it was potentially harmful and, in the case of drug overdose, that the amount taken was excessive.

The essential distinction is between those who commit suicide (completed suicide) and those who survive after harming themselves (parasuicide and self-harm). The challenge for the psychiatrist lies in that there is substantial overlap between the two.

Risk factors for suicide: features from the history that are associated with increased risk of suicide

The main risk factors are as follows:

- **Statement of intent:** about two-thirds of those who die by suicide have told someone about their intentions. It is a misconception that those who talk about suicide do not act upon it.
- **History of previous self-harm behaviour:** around 40 per cent of people presenting with self-harm have a history of at least one previous attempt. Around 20 per cent of all those who repeat, do so within 12 months of the first attempt.
- **Presence of psychiatric disorder:** over 90 per cent of those who complete suicide have a psychiatric disorder at the time of committing suicide. The prevalence of psychiatric disorders among self-harm cases is also very high. Those disorders with a higher risk of suicide are major depression, bipolar affective disorder, schizophrenia, and drug/alcohol dependence.

Further risk factors of suicide to remember and recognize are:
- painful physical illness
- bereavement
- impulsive personality traits
- social isolation
- male sex
- unemployment
- low social class
- older age (however, risk is increasing in young men)
- previous history of self-harm
- certain professions (doctors, veterinary surgeons, farmers)
- certain ethnic groups (Indian females).

Features associated with higher suicide risk
- recurrent or persisting suicidal ideation (always remember to ask)
- hopelessness
- depression
- agitation
- early schizophrenia with retained insight (young patients who are aware of the implications of their illness and see their future ambitions restricted)
- presence of delusions of control, poverty, and guilt
- being under the effects of alcohol or other substance (intoxication = decreased self-control = risk)
- personality trait of impulsivity.

The systematic risk assessment and management of suicide/self-harm
The assessment is aimed at identifying subjects at risk and estimating the chances of suicidal ideas leading to acts or of repetition of self-harm behaviour (Table 8.1). Prevention of repeated self-harm and completed suicide is the goal.
1. The patient recovering from self-harm needs to be physically stable before you conduct a psychiatric assessment. Assessment of drowsy patients after an overdose is unreliable.
2. A crucial step is routinely making tactful but direct inquiries about the patient's intentions. Asking about suicide does not make it more likely to happen.
3. An essential part of the assessment is to determine the presence of any psychiatric disorder, i.e. to obtain a full psychiatric history and conduct a thorough mental state examination (see Chapter 4).
4. All the risk factors discussed here need to be explored. There are scales to help to do this systematically and a flexible use of these is recommended (see the 'SAD PERSONS' Scale in Appendix 3).
5. Identify any precipitating factors. Ask about life events, conflicts in areas of relationships, employment, finances, law/police, housing, sexual adjustment, physical health, and bereavement. Precipitating factors need to be addressed/resolved if further risk is to be prevented or decreased.

Table 8.1 Features conveying higher risk of repetition and eventual suicide

Higher risk	Lower risk
Previous self-harm	First attempt
Attempt planned	Impulsive attempt (non-planned)
Attempt performed in isolation	Attempt performed in front of others
Precautions taken to avoid rescue	Rescue intervention is likely or actively sought
Violent method (hanging, gun)	Non-violent method (overdose)
Patient expected fatal outcome	Patient was unsure of outcome*
Regrets having been rescued	Relieved at being rescued
'Suicide note' or will written	No 'suicide note' or will written

* What matters are the patient's subjective intentions/expectations, irrespective of real medical seriousness.

6. It is also necessary to evaluate the degree of social support available to the patient and to assess previous coping strategies. Could the patient's family help? Involvement of the patient's GP should be routine practice.
7. Finally, if in doubt, always consult a more experienced colleague.

When these key aspects are fully explored, a management plan will be established, the principles of which are as follows:

- In patients judged to be at low repetition risk and with no major mental illness, the principles of **crisis intervention** apply: 'understand' the attempt; mobilize resources; consider a 'non-self-harm' contract; discharge preferably to relatives; inform GP; consider referral to a service able to offer some form of psychotherapeutic intervention and a point of contact.
- In patients judged to be a high repetition risk, with major mental illness, admission needs to be considered, with a MHA assessment as necessary. Community management depends on the local resources available (e.g. home treatment team, supportive relatives, GP, community psychiatric nurse).
- In patients who frequently repeat, the same principles apply; a long-term management plan involving a psychological framework and consistency of contact needs to be established to prevent counterproductive care.
- Risk can never be excluded completely and suicide remains stubbornly difficult to predict; careful note-taking and interdisciplinary communication are vital for your patient's health and your own legal protection. When psychiatrists' interventions successfully prevent suicides, no proof of efficacy exists, and often there is no acknowledgement; however, a completed suicide can be seen as a professional failure. This irony of our profession is also a source of legal activity.

Alcohol and drug use

Alcohol and drug use is common among people with psychiatric illness, and people who use drugs or drink heavily are at higher risk of developing psychiatric problems. Thus, assessment of drug and alcohol use should form part of all psychiatric assessments. If initial screening suggests problems, then a more thorough history should be taken. Although people with chronic relapsing substance dependence can engender feelings of 'therapeutic despair', it should be borne in mind that the majority of people who develop drug- or alcohol-related problems do recover. Provided appropriate and realistic goals are set, facilitating change in this patient group can be very rewarding.

Assessment of people with drug and alcohol problems involves more than just information gathering; allowing the patient time to tell their story offers an opportunity for reflection, and the initial therapeutic engagement may influence the course of their treatment. The patient may have previous experiences of rejection or criticism from public services, and a non-judgemental, collaborative approach may increase their likelihood of returning for treatment. When introducing the drug and alcohol history, a general invitation such as 'Tell me about your drug use' or 'What role does drinking have in your life?' may elicit more honest and informative responses than an immediate focus on precise quantities and frequencies. Keep in mind the main aims of your assessment: to distinguish between use, harmful use, and dependence; to identify comorbidities, risks, and harms; and to explore motivation for change.

Important elements of the history

- Which substances is the patient using?
- What is the frequency of use?
- What is the pattern of a typical drug-using day or week?
- What is the route of use (e.g. oral, smoked, snorted, injected)?
- What effect is the patient seeking?
- Is there evidence of the physical or psychological features of dependence?
- What risky behaviours does the patient engage in (e.g. injecting, sharing needles, unsafe sex, 'sex for drugs')?
- How long is the history of drug use and how has it evolved?
- What complications of drug use has the patient experienced (physical, psychological, family, occupational, and legal problems)?
- What is the patient's past experience of treatment for a drug problem? Have there been any periods of abstinence and, if so, what has helped the patient to achieve this? What triggers have brought on relapses?

Current use

Enquire about amounts used and frequency. Ask also about the circumstances of use; for example, some people will only use drugs in certain social circumstances, such as ecstasy use at a dance party, while others may have a regular pattern of use that has developed to prevent the experience of withdrawal symptoms. For alcohol, check the brand or strength: beer and cider can vary from 3 per cent to 9.5 per cent alcohol concentration.

Prescription drugs can usually be assessed by dose. For illicit drugs, the amount of money spent may give a reasonable approximation. Be aware of uncertainties around amounts/purity: liquid preparations may be diluted, tablets passed off as other drugs, and powders/rocks may be heavily cut with other psychoactive or inactive substances.

Obtain alcohol consumption (units) for the past 24 hours, 6 months, and 12 months (1 unit = 8–10 g of alcohol which is equivalent to one glass of wine, half a pint of ordinary strength beer, or one measure of spirits).

Club drugs, stimulants, and 'legal highs'

A large number of newly-synthesized drugs, derived from known psychotropic drugs, are regularly released in an attempt to circumvent drug laws. These are increasingly available by mail order via the internet. The precise substances are too many and varied to list here, so general enquiry into the use of any other substances should be made. Particular drugs of note are GBL (gamma-hydroxybutyrolactone), which can be associated with accidental overdose and rapid severe dependence, methamphetamine, and mephedrone.

A typical day

Enquiring about a typical 24-hour period helps assess patterns of use in an open way. Patients with large variability in alcohol and drug use may have a tendency to bingeing and can be asked about light days, heavy days, and any brief periods of abstinence. Ask the patient to take you through the day from the moment of waking, including usual activities, work, social contact, and interests as well as drug and alcohol use. A description of the timing and intensity of any withdrawal symptoms, consumption of first drink or drugs, and the patient's attitude towards it, can be helpful in determining the degree of dependence. Ask him/her to finish their description of the day by enquiring about sleep and insomnia, including the use of substances to aid sleep or use during the night to relieve withdrawal symptoms. A man waking at 4.00 a.m., tremulous and drenched in sweat, who reaches out for the can of strong beer by the bed, is at a different stage of dependence from the man who takes his first drink at lunch time. Likewise, the professional woman who binges on cocaine every week is at a different stage from the woman whose daily routine revolves around obtaining enough money through illicit means to keep cocaine withdrawal symptoms at bay. Enquiring about patterns of use over the last week may give additional information.

Features of dependence

Note the presence and age of onset of withdrawal symptoms and other features of the dependence syndrome (ICD-10): compulsion to drink/use, difficulties in controlling amount taken, tolerance, progressive neglect of alternative pleasures or interests, persistent use despite clear evidence of harmful consequences.

History of drug use

In addition to current drug use, ask the patient if s/he has used other drugs in the past. If the patient has used more than one drug, it is usually easier to take a chronological history of each drug in turn rather than to try to assess all of them at once.

Ask about the age at first use, and then when the patient began to increase frequency of use. Ask about maximum frequency and amount used, and about any periods of abstinence. Also enquire about the social context at different stages, e.g. in a group, alone in a social setting, or alone at home. When (if ever) did the patient first experience withdrawal symptoms? Ask the patient to describe them.

Harms and complications

Outline physical, psychological, and social problems and risk-taking behaviour.

Physical problems associated with alcohol

GI: gastritis, hepatitis, cirrhosis, pancreatitis, peptic ulcer, oesophageal varices, oesophageal carcinoma.

Neuropsychiatric: seizures, cognitive impairment, peripheral neuropathy, cerebellar degeneration, delirium tremens, Wernicke's encephalopathy, alcoholic hallucinosis, memory blackouts, pathological intoxication.

Other: anaemia, cardiomyopathy, myopathy, head injury, etc.

Physical complications associated with injecting drug use

Abscesses, pneumonia, deep vein thromboses, endocarditis, septicaemia, collapsed veins. Ask about risky injecting behaviour, e.g. injecting into groin, neck, or infected injection sites, sharing needles or injecting paraphernalia ('works'). Ask specifically about hepatitis B, C, and HIV and immunization history (e.g. 'Have you ever worried that you might have caught hepatitis? Or HIV? Have you had any tests?').

Psychological complications

Ask about the relationship of psychological symptoms to alcohol and drug use. It may be difficult to tease out cause and effect, but some initial information will help in your assessment. Consider depression, anxiety, suicide attempts, pathological jealousy, personality change, sexual dysfunction, eating disorders.

Sexual and relationship problems

Ask about sexual problems; STD risk behaviour; marital/relationship problems related to drinking or drug use; separation; domestic violence (as a victim or perpetrator, or both); divorce; problems with children.

Social and legal problems

Assess the extent to which the patient's main social contacts are other drug or alcohol users. Occupation working with alcohol (pubs or bars)? Work problems related to alcohol (dismissal, absenteeism, frequent job changes). Debts (e.g. rent arrears, unpaid credit cards bills, money owed to dealers). Ask about how s/he is financing the alcohol or drug use. Forensic history— drug use offences, acquisitive crime, drink–driving offences. Ask about any outstanding court cases.

Treatment history

Any successful periods of abstinence without assistance? Help from services e.g. GP, community addiction team (statutory or voluntary); planned detoxes (e.g. in specialist addiction unit); unplanned detoxes (e.g. when admitted with a medical emergency); residential rehabilitation; self-help group (Alcoholics Anonymous, Narcotics Anonymous). Duration of any periods of abstinence. What does the patient think was helpful in the past? What influences have helped the patient to achieve abstinence and then later to relapse?

Current goals and motivations

Abstinence is one possible goal, but safer use may be a more realistic inter-mediate goal (see Chapter 9, 'Alcohol and drug misuse', p. 144). Many patients do not identify the drug/alcohol use as the main issue but are seek-ing help with mood issues, relationship problems, etc. Ask the patient what s/he sees as the priority and what s/he would like to do about the drug/alcohol use. Motivation may be assessed by asking two questions: how *important* it is to make a change, and how *confident* the patient is of making that change.

Background history

This should be the same as for any psychiatric history. The personal his-tory and premorbid personality (what s/he was like before developing his/her drinking/drug problem) is important to clarify. Particular elements of the medical, psychiatric, forensic, and social history have already been highlighted.

Physical examination

- Physical signs of withdrawal.
- Alcohol-related problems: nystagmus, ophthalmoplegia, ataxia, peripheral neuropathy, tremor, dysdiadochokinesis, hepatomegaly, signs of liver disease, bruising.
- Look for injection sites, including legs and groins. If the patient is injecting, ask him or her to show you the most recent injection sites. Look for abscesses or infected sinuses, and for evidence of deep vein thrombosis.

Investigations

FBC, U&E, LFT, HIV and hepatitis screening. ECG for people on >100 mg methadone/day (risk of QT prolongation).

Eating disorders

History

Many sufferers from eating disorders feel ashamed about what they are doing and may find your questions very taxing and painful. Others are ambivalent about whether they want help; in some cases, the denial is so extreme that they feel that there is little or nothing wrong with them and have merely come to the clinic because of the excessive concerns of their family or partner. Particularly in these latter cases, it is important to estab-lish an individual relationship with the patient rather than to relate exclu-sively to the family.

Patients are typically female (ratio 10:1). They arouse strong feelings, ranging from anger and irritation through to the desire to rescue and protect. This is probably because their interpersonal schemas include a mixture of a drive to please others, a sense of inferiority, and a drive to be in control. One of the most important parts of the management is to understand these relationship dynamics, both for therapeutic purposes and because they may affect clinical judgement.

Behavioural assessment

At the simplest level, the clinician wants to know the following by the end of the assessment interview:

• Is there severe undernutrition or significant overweight?
• Is there constant dietary restriction and/or are there episodes of overeating?
• What weight control measures are used?

These behavioural criteria are easy to define and elicit, but they are also of clinical utility as they guide management.

Undernutrition or overweight?

This is addressed by measuring weight and height, and is usually done at the end of the interview with the physical examination (see following details). A detailed lifetime weight and diet history is helpful. The patient should be asked when s/he first noticed a problem with her/his weight or when s/he first began to focus on weight as a topic of personal importance. Both the **rate** of weight loss and the **absolute level** are crucial when assessing clinical risk. Marked fluctuations suggest that there is self-induced vomiting or abuse of laxatives and diuretics.

  The patient should be asked what her/his heaviest ever weight was and when this occurred, and similarly about their lowest weight. The weight at which periods began needs to be established, as does the weight at which periods stopped (if relevant). This is important, as the weight at which a patient's normal biological functions recover will generally be slightly above the former and so can give an indication of how much weight needs to be gained.

  It is also useful to obtain a family weight history. There may be a strong family history of obesity in bulimia nervosa, or of leanness or eating disorder in anorexia nervosa.

Constant dietary restriction and/or episodes of overeating?

It is often necessary to question directly about bulimic behaviour as it may not be spontaneously mentioned because of the shame attached. A suitable line of enquiry is 'Do you have episodes when your eating seems excessive or out of control?'. You need to probe gently to elicit whether the amount eaten is excessive (objective binge, >1000 kcal) or not (subjective binge).

What weight control measures are used?

In addition to dietary restriction, the methods commonly employed are self-induced vomiting, chewing, and spitting; abuse of laxatives, diuretics, street drugs (e.g. amphetamines and ecstasy), caffeine, prescribed medication such as thyroxine, or health food preparations; and excessive exercise.

Mental state assessment

Overvalued ideas about shape and weight, in which the assessment of self-worth is made exclusively in these terms, are considered primary features of bulimia nervosa. Not all patients with anorexia nervosa express such ideas.

Body image distortion (a statement that they are fat when they are underweight) is no longer regarded as a necessary criterion for anorexia nervosa. A less culturally bound description of this phenomenon is that the emaciated state is overvalued.

The patient should also be asked what weight s/he would ideally like to be. Often, patients with anorexia nervosa will try to please the therapist by giving a higher weight than they are aiming for. It may be helpful to probe into this in some detail: 'If you got to seven stone would you be happy there?'. If the patient says 'no', it can be helpful to press her/him as this may help her/him realize that there is a problem: 'So if you were seven stone, you might want to weigh six and a half, but what then?'.

Additional psychiatric disorders

Over 80 per cent of subjects with eating disorders have additional psychiatric morbidity during the course of their life. Depression and obsessional symptoms are common in anorexia nervosa. Depression and anxiety disorders are common in bulimia. Symptoms of post-traumatic stress disorder are common in mixed anorexia nervosa and bulimia nervosa. Personality disorders are present in half of cases referred to specialist centres.

Diagnostic features to look out for are:
- body mass index (BMI) less than 17.5 kg/m²
- use of weight control measures
- physical signs such as parotid or submandibular gland enlargement, eroded teeth, 'Russell's sign' callus on back of hand, cold blue hands, lanugo hair.

BMI can be calculated as follows:

$$BMI = weight (kg) / [height (m)]^2$$

Factors for converting from imperial to metric measures and vice versa are given in Table 8.2.

Physical assessment

Nutrition

Many patients find it very difficult to allow themselves to be weighed. It is important not to be drawn into a battle over this. In general, the higher the weight, the more lenient you can afford to be. The ICD-10 definition of anorexia nervosa requires that the BMI is less than 17.5 kg/m².

Table 8.2 Conversion of imperial and metric measures for weight and height

	Imperial to metric	Metric to imperial
Weight	1 stone = 6.35 kg	1 kg = 0.16 stone
	1 lb = 0.45 kg	1 kg = 2.2 lb
Height	1 ft = 30.5 cm	1 m = 3.3 ft
	1 in = 2.54 cm	1 cm = 0.39 in

1 stone = 14 lb; 1 ft = 12 in; 1 m = 100 cm.

Cardiovascular system

The hands, feet, and nose are pinched, blue, and cold. In severe cases, chilblains and, particularly in children, gangrene of the toes can occur. The heart rate is slow (<60 beats/min) and blood pressure is low (90/60 mmHg). A marked fall in blood pressure on standing (postural drop) is evidence of dehydration.

Skin and hair

The skin is dry and downy, and lanugo hair may be present on the cheeks, the nape of the neck, and the forearms and legs. The head hair may become thinned and dry so that it breaks off and sticks out. There may be a scar over the knuckles (Russell's sign) if the hand is used to induce vomiting. A petechial rash due to thrombocytopenia can occur with severe starvation.

Gastrointestinal system

Vomiting can lead to many physical consequences. The teeth may appear small and smooth, with the upper front teeth worn into an arch shape; alternatively, the teeth may be deceptively even as if they have been crowned. The side of the mouth may be cracked. The face may appear rounded because of swelling of the salivary glands.

Skeletomuscular system

In severe cases, a proximal myopathy develops. If this is present, the patient may find it difficult to lift her/his arms to brush their hair. S/he may not be able to get up without help or without arm leverage if you ask her/him to crouch. Tetany can develop because of the metabolic alkalosis (common in vomiting).

Management

Anorexia nervosa

Outpatient psychotherapy is the recommended treatment for the majority of people with anorexia nervosa Specialist psychotherapies such as cognitive analytical therapy, cognitive–behavioural therapy, family therapy, interpersonal therapy, or modified dynamic therapy are more effective than non-specialist or dietetic treatment. Frequently, the therapy has to be continued long term. It is important that this is supplemented by regular medical monitoring. It is helpful to have the patient's family involved in treatment. Parental counselling is as effective and more acceptable to the family than conjoint family therapy.

Inpatient treatment is necessary for those with severe weight loss and high medical risk. Staff with expertise in management of eating disorders can provide a judicious mixture of psychotherapy and nutritional support. In extreme circumstances, people may be detained under the Mental Health Act.

Bulimia nervosa

Cognitive behavioural therapy (16–20 sessions) is the treatment of choice for the majority of patients with bulimia nervosa. Low-intensity interventions such as self-help with guidance, group treatment, or antidepressant therapy may be useful as a first step in treatment for a proportion of cases, especially those with less severe symptoms. Patients with comorbid personality disorders or with additional physical morbidity, such as diabetes mellitus, may need long-term psychotherapy, inpatient care, or day care.

Treatment must address the psychological aspects of anorexia and bulimia nervosa as well as the eating behaviour. Re-feeding alone may be successful in short-term weight restoration but is usually not effective in the long term.

Investigations recommended on initial assessment

- Full blood count (cells reduced: white cell count > red blood cells > platelets)
- Urea and electrolytes (low potassium, magnesium, calcium, and phosphate; high bicarbonate)
- Liver function test (all enzymes raised, severe starvation) and protein (decrease rare but sign of poor prognosis)
- ECG (QT lengthening, U wave).

Somatization

Somatization is the expression of emotional distress in physical terms, with medical help seeking. At interview, most of these patients will fulfil diagnostic criteria for a psychological disorder (usually depression and/or anxiety), but will often deny that they have an emotional problem. This is a very common presentation of psychological disorder and is neither abnormal nor unusual.

It is essential that such patients are physically examined and receive any appropriate investigations. When results are fed back to the patient, it is important to acknowledge that the physical symptoms are real and do not suggest, either directly or by implication, that the patient is 'nervous' or is exaggerating the symptoms. Instead, s/he is reminded of the other psychological symptoms that are present, and the presenting symptoms are 'reframed'. The way is then clear to explain the mechanisms by which emotional distress can cause physical symptoms.

Somatization disorder refers to the most severe cases, and is a diagnostic category to describe patients who report large numbers of somatic symptoms, have illness histories stretching back to adolescence, and are very frequent users of medical services. The disorder is uncommon, but is very demanding in terms of cost and time.

Taking a history from a patient with severe somatization can be difficult if one is a psychiatrist. The intention is to obtain the usual information on the mental state, but without challenging the patient or becoming too 'psychological'. Thus, do not ask 'Are you depressed?' but 'Has all this got you down?'; do not ask 'Do you feel like killing yourself?' but 'Have all your problems ever got too much for you?'; and so on. Do not ask 'Do you get panic attacks?' but, instead, probe about whether or not certain situations, such as supermarkets or the tube, make the patient worse. The patient who tells you that s/he is made worse by neon lights, or whose 'brain gets overloaded by lots of conversations going on at once', may be experiencing phobic-related symptoms. Stress is a term that is often acceptable to patients when more direct psychological approaches fail.

One of the most important questions is 'What do you think is wrong with you?'. The patient's illness model may explain much of his/her behaviour, as well as pointing to possible treatment avenues. Someone who is worried that when s/he has back pain, his/her 'disk will slip again' and s/he will end up in a wheelchair, will naturally restrict their activities. Many have similar 'catastrophic' cognitions: 'If I push myself, I may never walk again, or I'll have a relapse'. Always ask 'What might happen if you continued [when you get the pain/feel exhausted/feel dizzy]?' and 'What is the worst thing that might happen to you?'.

History

The medical and family history of patients with chronic somatization can be revealing. A history of previous unexplained symptoms is common: tonsillitis persisting after the removal of tonsils, 'grumbling appendix', prolonged recovery from normal infections, repeated gynaecological procedures, and so on. Illness may also run in the family; looking after parents with long-term illnesses (either physical or psychological) is common. Previous episodes of ill-defined illnesses, such as candida or unusual allergies, are suggestive.

Always take a history of previous contacts with the medical profession. It is not advisable to criticize medical colleagues, but allow the patient to ventilate his/her distress at what may have been very unsatisfactory previous encounters.

Course

Subacute somatization is very common and the physical symptoms are likely to remit eventually. However, if the patient receives an endless series of negative physical investigations, it is only a matter of time before s/he develops a chronic form of somatization disorder. Patients attending specialist clinics with labels such as myalgic encephalomyelitis (ME) or chronic fatigue syndrome also have a gloomy outlook, associated with the strength of their physical illness convictions and the degree of avoidance behaviour.

Investigations

In general, most patients with somatization disorder will already have had more than enough investigations. Once basic sensible investigations have been performed, further investigations will reinforce the sense that something organic is wrong. Investigations do not reassure such patients, and induce anxiety rather than relieving it. A better use of your time is to obtain as many medical records as you can.

Management

Management has several purposes: first, to engage the patient in some form of dialogue; secondly, to reduce further doctor visits and medical investigations: thirdly, if possible, to treat any underlying psychological disorder. It is essential that the patient feels understood; listen to the whole history of the symptoms and their impact. You are not taking a history for diagnostic purposes, but so that the patient feels that you have listened and understood his/her predicament and suffering.

Supportive psychotherapy involves seeing the patient regularly, but not in response to symptoms. Rather than saying 'Come and see me when you feel bad', say 'Come every month anyway'. Each session usually involves listening to some account of the symptoms and their impact, even if you can do nothing about them. It is useful to split the session in two, spending the first half talking about symptoms and health, and then allowing the patient to set another agenda incorporating coping strategies.

More specific techniques, usually following cognitive–behavioural principles, are valuable. These often involve some combination of cognitive work, looking at explanations for symptoms, generating alternative explanations, and examining the links between sleep, mood, illness fears, and symptoms. This may be followed by some form of activity management programme with the intention of reducing the link between the experience of symptoms and some maladaptive behaviour pattern (such as going to bed). It is useful to give sensible explanations for symptoms so that patients have an understanding of why they experience them and do not feel that you believe their symptoms are imaginary. Explaining the role of muscle tension in headache or chest pain, anxiety in palpitations, poor sleep and daytime fatigue, inactivity in muscle pain, and hyperventilation in breathlessness and chest pain can all be useful.

Symptom checklists may be useful both to monitor progress and, if planning to try an antidepressant, to check that any reported side-effects really are new. The guiding principle is to empower patients to take back responsibility for their illness and recovery (and not rely on doctors, drugs, surgical procedures, etc.), but without harbouring any guilt or blame for becoming ill in the first place. This is harder than it sounds.

Things not to do

If the patient has a specific illness belief ('candida', 'ME', 'chronic allergy'), do not question this, even if there is no corroborating medical evidence. Do not dispute the condition by saying 'This illness doesn't exist!'. Instead, accept the label and move on to 'How can we help you live with the symptoms/distress?' or 'How can we help you reduce your pain/disability?'. Never attempt to switch the patient from a wholly physical to a solely psychological model. This is both inappropriate and largely impossible. Once you have checked that basic investigations have been performed (such as routine biochemical/haematological screen and thyroid function tests), do not refer for more specialist opinions or tests unless some new indication, suggestive of a physical cause, comes along.

Pharmacological management

Depression and anxiety are often present and need treatment. There is some evidence that low-dose tricyclics can be effective where pain and sleep problems coexist. Many patients are reluctant to take antidepressants, but may accept them on these grounds.

Response to treatment

Most patients with somatization are seen in primary care, are easy to engage with, and respond well to simple treatments. Cognitive–behavioural treatments are successful in those with discrete disorders such as atypical chest pain, chronic fatigue, or low back pain. However, those with long histories, who may fulfil criteria for somatization disorder, have a poor prognosis.

Limiting the expectations of a cure and concentrating on maximizing function by 'damage limitation', through support and encouragement, may be all that one can achieve.

Mother and baby problems

Pregnancy

At some time or another, most general psychiatrists will look after female patients who are pregnant, and a detailed assessment of the mother's mental health and adjustment may be necessary for a variety of purposes or the reasons listed here. Maternal psychopathology in pregnancy is the same as psychopathology in other settings, and thus the principles of detailed history taking and systematic mental state evaluation are the same, irrespective of childbearing status. However, the interviewer should be sensitive to the fact that, in general, only a fortunate few expectant mothers conform to the stereotype of the pregnant woman who 'blooms' with good health, and for many mothers, early pregnancy is a time of tiredness, appetite changes, nausea, loss of libido, etc. There may be anxieties and concerns about the future, doubts about readiness for parenthood, and uncertainties about the stability of key relationships (e.g. with the partner). Fears, ruminations, and fantasies about the fetus may have a bearing on the mother's mental state, but may not be mentioned unless asked about, and then only if the mother has confidence in the interviewer.

What is the personal and social context of the pregnancy? Is it a first baby? Have there been previous miscarriages and terminations? If it is a second or subsequent pregnancy, how old are the other children? Are they in good health? Is the mother anticipating problems with the arrival of the new child? How much help and support does she have from family and friends, and how supportive is the expectant father financially, practically, and emotionally? What is his mental health like? Thus, the context of pregnancy imparts a particular focus to the psychiatric examination, and in terms of the mother's history, it becomes especially important to know what her own experience of being parented was like and what experience she has had of looking after babies and little children.

Clinically significant depression and anxiety is not uncommon in early pregnancy and may be missed unless specifically asked about. Clinical judgement is needed to distinguish between psychosomatic concomitants of depression and changes that occur in pregnancy. For example, can a woman who wakes up at night to micturate go back to sleep easily? Does she wake feeling refreshed? Is there a diurnal variation to her tiredness and is her loss of appetite specific to certain kinds of foods? How does *she* construe her physical symptoms, i.e. does she ascribe them to her pregnant condition?

Some important reasons for psychiatric examination in pregnancy

Termination of pregnancy

Abortion legislation varies greatly across nations and it is not possible to generalize about psychiatric indications. Suicidal risk and the possibility of severe postpartum destabilization of mental health are among the most prominent psychiatric considerations in countries with relatively restrictive abortion laws. There are no *absolute* psychiatric indications or contraindications to abortion; that is, apart from religious, moral, and legal considerations, there are no psychiatric illnesses or indeed associated disorders (e.g. severe mental impairment) in which a woman's right to choose may be overruled on medical/psychiatric grounds.

Management of severe mental illness during pregnancy

Questions often arise about the teratogenic effects of prescribed and non-prescribed drugs. What balance is there between the putative benefits of discontinuing medication and a flare-up of maternal illness? Clearly, such questions can only be addressed in the light of a detailed knowledge of the mother's history and current state.

Welfare of the fetus; future safety of parenting of the newborn

Risks to the fetus may arise through infection, nutritional deficit, drug exposure, deliberate self-harm, and lack of compliance with antenatal care programmes. Thus, the assessment of the mother's condition (e.g. chronic schizophrenia, eating disorder, drug dependence, personality disorder, depression, mental impairment) takes on an added urgency because of the risk to the unborn child, and this risk may enter the equation when assessing the need for compulsory treatment under the provisions of the Mental Health Act. Longer-term concerns about motivation and safety of parenting of the newborn should begin to be addressed during pregnancy, in conjunction with social services. The psychiatrist may be asked to carry out an evaluation of the mother's mental illness, its history and prognosis, and her ability to manage her life in her personal and social context. There may be an inherent conflict between the mother's rights and wishes to be the primary carer of her baby and the paramount need to ensure the child's welfare and safety.

Prevention and management of postpartum recurrence

The likelihood of recurrence of severe mental illness (manic depressive and schizoaffective disorder, and possibly also paranoid psychosis) is high. Relapse rates of up to 50 per cent are described, and therefore it is negligent not to plan ahead by liaising with obstetric and primary health care services and planning possible admission. Recurrence rates of non-psychotic depressive disorders are about 20 per cent, and if a woman is taking an antidepressant medication, and discontinues it, the recurrence rates can be as high as 70 per cent, especially when the medication is discontinued abruptly. Accurate and expert antenatal assessment by a psychiatrist is essential for planned management at a time when the mother is in repeated contact with clinical (obstetric and primary health care) services. Motivation to change may be a major factor in helping some expectant mothers to alter patterns of behaviour (e.g. drug use and abuse).

After childbirth

The same general principles that applied to psychiatric examination in pregnancy also apply after the birth of the child. Thus, some kinds of pre-existing mental illness have high rates of recurrence, but in addition, childbirth itself is a major factor in provoking first onsets of both psychotic and non-psychotic affective disorder. There are three conditions, the names of which suggest a specific association with childbirth: maternity blues, postnatal depression, and postpartum or puerperal psychosis.

Maternity blues

These are near universal, short-lived episodes of emotional lability, typically occurring around the fourth and fifth days postpartum. The most common picture is of dysphoria, but this may, in some instances, be mingled with or dominated by elation, prolixity, and overactivity. The blues themselves do not constitute an illness or syndrome, and the two main points of clinical interest are the identification of the characteristics of those women who go on to develop postnatal depression, and the distinction between the 'benign' self-limiting mood changes of the blues from the sinister prodromal symptoms of impending affective psychosis.

Postnatal depression

The symptoms of postnatal depression are the same as those of depression in other settings but, in addition, the women frequently report ruminations of inadequacy and guilt about their ability to be good or competent mothers. Sometimes, they describe feelings of aggression and impulses to harm the infant, which are very rarely acted upon but which induce further self-blame. Thus, the assessment of depression after childbirth should always incorporate sensitive questions about the mother's feelings concerning her baby, and should extend to include obsessional ruminations and rituals as well as psychological and behavioural manifestations of anxiety (e.g. irrational fears, social and agoraphobic behaviours). Women suffering from postnatal depression may struggle to bond with their infant, thus jeopardizing the early attachment process and harming the infant's psychological development and well-being.

Postpartum or puerperal psychosis

These are affective (manic, mixed, or psychotic depressive) disorders, sometimes with paranoid hallucinatory symptoms as well, which have an acute onset, usually at the end of the first or during the second week after delivery. There may be a 'lucid' period of a few days, and the affective illness often fluctuates, with rapid mood swings. In addition, it is suggested that the presence of 'non-organic' confusion (i.e. perplexity and patchy disorientation) may be pathognomonic.

The choice of drugs is based on a judgement of the predominant clinical picture. Repeated assessments may be necessary, and too frequent changes of medication leading to polypharmacy should be avoided. Such assessments should also take into account possible risks to the infant if mother and baby are admitted together to a specialist Mother and Baby Unit. Risks may arise in response to hallucinations or delusions, for example, that the baby is evil and possessed, or is highly critical of the new mother, or is immortal, or is an angel. Another major source of risk is through disorganization and neglect because the mother's interactions are too disturbed, for example, because she is manic or agitated. Her interactions may be diminished because of psychomotor retardation, or they may be inappropriate because she is chronically and severely impaired and lacking insight as part of a schizophrenic illness. In such circumstances, the psychiatric examination must synthesize your own evaluation of the mother's mental state (including behaviour) both alone and in the presence of the baby, with the observations of nurses and other members of the clinical team.

Decisions about whether, temporarily, to nurse mother and baby separately may have to be backed by compulsion under the provisions of the Mental Health Act. Similarly, the decision about when it is safe to reunite them must depend upon the psychiatrist's assessment of the mother's mental state, her awareness of illness, and her adherence, with necessary restrictions. The baby's father (or person who shares parental responsibility), the family, or possibly social services will be involved in this decision.

Learning disabilities

People with learning disabilities are more vulnerable to mental health or behavioural problems. Detection of psychiatric disorders can be problematic and diagnoses may be missed. Assessment of mental state requires modification of approaches used for people without learning disabilities, with particular emphasis on appropriate means of communication.

People with learning disabilities may be distressed for a number of reasons, including pain and physical health problems, abuse, and bereavement, and it is important to consider these as part of the psychiatric assessment.

The history

As in all psychiatric assessments, a full history is an essential component to the assessment. The interviewer will have asked about presenting complaints, the history of the problem, physical health (including epilepsy), and past psychiatric history. It is also important to understand recent life events, daily living skills and activities, level of support, and relationships. Personal history should be considered, including a developmental history, details of schooling and educational achievements, and family history. The role of the family and carers should be discussed.

Informant information should always be sought as people with learning disability might have limitations in recalling the chronology of events.

The mental state examination

There are specific issues and adaptations to consider in the mental state examination.

General considerations
- Access to previous reports/information.
- Informant information is important in order to consider recent changes in behaviour.
- An unfamiliar environment might alter the person's behaviour. Assessment in a familiar setting should be considered.
- Communication may be limited. Alternative styles of communication should be considered including Maketon (a sign language developed for people with learning disabilities) and PECS (using pictures and diagrams as a means of communication).

Appearance and behaviour
- Observation of behaviour over a period of time is important, particularly in non-verbal patients.

Speech/communication
- Consider how the person usually communicates with others.
- Articulation defects might make understanding problematic—an informant might be helpful as an 'interpreter'.

Mood
- Features of depression might include a reduction in engagement in usual activities.
- Hypomanic/manic symptoms are not dissimilar to those in people without learning disabilities.
- In those with autism, mood disorders might be displayed as an exaggeration of usual behaviours.

Thought content
- Autistic beliefs and preoccupations can mimic psychotic belief and experiences.
- People with learning disabilities are suggestible. Always try to use open questions.
- Drawings might be helpful when communicating thought content.

Cognition
- A deterioration in cognitive functioning should be considered.
- Behaviours should be interpreted in the light of the cognitive level.

Insight
- In those with mild/moderate learning disability, insight should always be assessed. People with severe/profound learning disability are unlikely to understand their mental health needs.

Other things to consider
- safeguarding
- consent and capacity.

Specific developmental disorders

These occur when there is an impairment of one or more developmental functions that is markedly out of keeping with the general level of development. For some functions, there are reliable and valid tests that have norms for different ages; for example, specific reading retardation occurs when performance on a standard reading test is worse than the fifth centile allowing for age and IQ, and it should be diagnosed by a psychologist's quantitative assessment. For other mental abilities (e.g. calculating), norms are much less satisfactory. For others again, such as motor delays and impairments of memory and attention, the diagnosis still has to be made on the basis of the clinical assessment. Remedial education can be given for all these problems, once the problem is recognized. Counselling for the child and family may be needed to help in the prevention of secondary psychiatric dysfunction. (See Chapter 3, 'Assessment of children with developmental disorders', p. 53.)

Management

The management of people with learning disabilities and mental health or behavioural problems generally involves a number of professionals and agencies.

Acute psychiatric or behavioural disturbance, in which the individual and/or others are placed at risk, demands prompt assessment and careful consideration of the most appropriate environment in which to manage the situation. Infrequently, hospital admission will be indicated. If this is the case, consideration should be given as to whether the person has the capacity to consent to an admission, or not; appropriate use of the Mental Health Act vs the Mental Capacity Act will form part of the initial assessment.

Hospital is not a long-term option and the aim should always be to manage people with learning disabilities and mental health problems in the community with appropriate multi-agency support.

Depending on the nature of the disorder, the following interventions will play a greater or lesser role in the management plan.

Psychosocial interventions

Behavioural disturbance should be assessed by professionals skilled in functional assessment. This enables the team working with the individual to understand reasons for the behaviour and consider whether these can be addressed. Examples would be difficulties in communicating needs or wishing to avoid certain situations.

An understanding of the person's cognitive level assists in ensuring that expectations and demands are appropriate.

Biological interventions

Medication may be indicated for specific psychiatric disorders including depression, anxiety, cyclical mood disorder, and psychosis.

Rapid tranquillization in the acute situation should only be considered as a last resort. People with learning disabilities can be very sensitive to sedative medication and can exhibit idiosyncratic side-effects. This should be used under strict medical supervision with resuscitation equipment available.

In the case of challenging behaviours where no clear psychiatric disorder is evident, psychological interventions should always be the first line of management. If psychological approaches alone are unsuccessful, or if the behaviour is presenting a very serious risk to self or others, then psychotropic medication might be indicated. The aim would be to use this to reduce arousal and agitation whilst continuing with behavioural strategies.

Conclusions

- People with learning disabilities are more vulnerable to developing psychiatric disorders.
- Assessment is complicated by communication difficulties.
- Assessment takes time and might need to be offered over a number of sessions.
- Informants should contribute to the assessment process.
- Management follows a bio-psycho-social model.
- Medication should be used with caution.

Epilepsy

Epileptic seizures

Epilepsy is the tendency for recurrent seizures and implies underlying brain disease. A single seizure or seizures occurring during acute medical illness is not epilepsy. Epileptic seizures are classified by onset into generalized or focal (clinical and EEG information facilitates this distinction).

Generalized epilepsy

- Generalized tonic-clonic ('grand mal') seizures, absence ('petit mal') seizures, and others (myoclonic seizures, atonic seizures). Generalized tonic-clonic seizures frequently occur without warning and involve loss of consciousness, usually for 1–10 minutes, and a phase of deep sleep from which the patient awakes often with a bitten tongue, aching, and signs of incontinence. Absence seizures do not occur *de novo* in adults. They resemble blank/frozen periods.

Focal (partial) epilepsy with or without secondary generalization

- **Simple partial seizures**: may be sensory, motor, autonomic, or psychic. Consciousness is not impaired. Symptom patterns tend to be stereotyped and have localizing value. Auras vary in their complexity from discrete sensory experiences to complex ideation and emotion. They are abrupt in onset, intrusive, and experienced passively.
- **Complex partial seizures** ('psychomotor seizures'): may be fugues, automatisms, and twilight states. Consciousness is impaired at onset but not lost.

Epilepsy in childhood

History

Begin by asking for details of the **first attack** experienced by the child: age, circumstances, description, duration, how it was dealt with. Then obtain similar details about subsequent attacks.

Be careful to distinguish and obtain separate descriptions of all different kinds of attack. For each type of attack, probe regarding the following points.

Pre-ictal

Precipitating events

Are they due to physical causes (illness, fever, etc.) or psychological causes (any stress or disturbance)?

Timing

Do they occur at any particular time of day or night? How long after last meal, etc.?

Altered behaviour or mental state before fit

Is s/he irritable, restless, confused, apathetic, etc. minutes or hours before the attack?

Patient's activity at onset
Do they occur while asleep, on wakening, or in full consciousness? Are they precipitated by over-breathing, watching television, walking out into bright sun, or any other change?

Ictal
Aura
What are the patient's subjective warning experiences? Ask the child whether s/he knows that the seizure is coming and what s/he notices first (giddiness, noises, lights, smell, funny taste, inability to speak, feels frightened, etc.). If the child cannot describe this experience, s/he may be able to draw it.

Course
What is the first event noticed (noises, strange behaviour, cry, fall to ground, motionless stare, etc.)? How long do the seizures last?

Posture during attack
Does the child fall, go limp, remain standing, slump back in chair, etc.?

Movements
Which parts move? One side or both? Synchronous or not (e.g. turning of head or eyes, tonic stiffening movements, clonic jerking movements, restless or semipurposive behaviour, automatic or repetitive acts, fumbling, mouth movements)?

Spread (march) of movements
Where does the fit start? Does it spread anywhere?

Consciousness
Is the child totally unresponsive? Aware, but unable to talk? Fully conscious and talking?

Colour changes
Does the child become pale, flushed, or blue?

Autonomic effects
Does the child become hot and sweaty, cold and sweaty, salivating, etc.?

Incontinence
Is there any incontinence of urine or faeces?

Injury
Is the tongue bitten or any other injury sustained?

Post-ictal
After-effects
Do they return to normal immediately or go to sleep or become sleepy? Are they confused? Is there any weakness or paralysis of arms or legs? Clumsiness? Difficulty with speech? Change of behaviour or emotional state? Other symptoms (e.g. headache)? Vomiting?

Type of seizure
If not mentioned by parent, ask specifically regarding the following:
1. **Generalized convulsive seizures:** Are there ever attacks in which the child passes out completely? Are there movements of the arms or legs in any of these attacks (tonic–clonic or clonic–tonic–clonic)?

2. **Generalized absence seizures:** Is there ever a momentary blank spell in which the child seems to be out of touch for a moment but does not fall down, and for which there is no memory subsequently? Are there any movements at all whilst this is happening?
3. **Other generalized seizures:** Does the child ever make odd jerky movements (myoclonus)? Does s/he ever fall down suddenly without jerking or going stiff (drop attacks)?
4. **Simple partial seizures:** Are there any attacks in which there are movements of the arms or legs, but the child does not pass out or lose touch?
5. **Complex partial seizures:** Does the child ever have episodes in which s/he does not seem to be him/herself or does peculiar things?
6. **Reflex attacks:** Does the child know how to stop an attack coming on? Ask him/her privately if s/he knows how to make an attack start.

Treatment

Is this by family doctor or paediatrician? Which drugs are used in what doses? (Calculate dose/kg/day: does it fall within the recommended range?) What side-effects are there? Have blood levels been measured recently? What do the parents do during the attack?

Attitudes

Obtain parental attitude to the attacks. What did they think was happening during the first attack? What do they put them down to? What does the child put them down to?

Does the child have epilepsy?

• **Differential diagnosis** includes syncope, breath-holding attacks, sleep disorder, benign paroxysmal vertigo.
• **Non-epileptic seizures ('pseudo-seizures')** are more common in children who also have epileptic seizures.
• Remember that **Münchausen's by proxy** is not uncommon. Obtain the name of someone other than the parent who has witnessed an attack and who can be contacted (e.g. a schoolteacher).

Notes

1. Children who are suspected or known to have seizures need a complete physical examination.
2. If the child is asked to count to 100, hesitations may reveal brief absence seizures.
3. Starting anticonvulsants is a serious decision. If there is still doubt, after a detailed history, about whether the child has seizures, consider asking the child to hyperventilate for 3 minutes. In susceptible children, this procedure will induce absence seizures in most, and complex partial seizures in a proportion. If a good history of generalized convulsive seizures has been obtained, there is no point in doing this test. In view of the potential danger, this procedure should be carried out only under careful supervision, including the availability of drugs and equipment for the management of status epilepticus.

Epilepsy in adults

History

Ask the patient if s/he has had a blackout recently and when exactly? Obtain a description of the attack. This should include a description by the patient, complemented by a description from an informant who has witnessed the attack. The patient may have had more than one form of attack. Ask him/her to describe a typical attack from the beginning.

Pre-ictal

Can the patient (or close observer) predict when an attack will happen minutes/hours before it does? How? Change in mood (irritability, dysphoria)? Change in cognition (inattentiveness, confused behaviour)? Build-up of minor seizures (myoclonic jerks)? Do these features resolve once the attack has occurred?

The epileptic attack

The presence of aura indicates focal cortical onset and strongly suggests underlying brain damage or disease. Is there any immediate warning of the attack or does the patient lose consciousness abruptly? If there is a warning, how long does it last? Does it last long enough to take avoiding action? Auras rarely exceed 1 minute in duration. Enquire about the aura content. Alimentary (epigastric sensations) and psychic (*déja vu*, hallucinatory) auras suggest a temporal lobe focus. A sensorimotor 'march' suggests a primary sensorimotor cortical focus.

- Is consciousness lost suddenly or gradually?
- Is the patient completely unconscious or does s/he retain some awareness of what is going on around him/her? If so, what?

What was the patient told of how s/he was while unconscious? Does s/he fall or slump to the ground or is s/he able to maintain their posture? Is s/he perfectly still or does s/he make movements? If the latter, are the movements rhythmic or irregular? Which parts of the body are involved? Are they more marked on one side of the body than the other? Is there any spread or are they generalized from the beginning? Is there any initial rotation of the head/eyes to one side?

- How long does this phase last?
- If the patient retains posture:
  - do they carry out any automatism (coordinated movement: fumbling, searching, etc.)?
  - is there any tongue/lip/cheek biting or urinary incontinence?
- After the patient appears to regain consciousness, how are they:
  - confused, sleepy, delayed speech recovery, quick recovery?
- Are any other epileptic episodes described:
  - absences, myoclonic jerks?

Course

- When was the first seizure?
- When was the patient first investigated? What was the patient/family told? When was s/he first started on anticonvulsants? Past seizure frequency? Present seizure frequency?
- Seizure pattern: diurnal? Nocturnal (how is this recognized)? Both?

- Precipitating factors: stress? Menses? Photic stimulation (self-induced flicker effect, television, nightclub stroboscope)? Lack of sleep? Non-compliance with medication?
- Predisposing factors: family history of epilepsy? Difficult birth? Febrile fits during infancy? History of head injury, brain infection (meningitis, encephalitis)? Seizures following immunization?

Diagnostic features to look out for
Other diagnostic possibilities

- **Non-epileptic seizures**: atypical features of the seizure (opisthotonos, pelvic thrusting, thrashing limbs, resists examination).
- **Panic disorder**: preceded by hyperventilation, chest discomfort, peripheral paraesthesiae, carpopedal spasm.
- **Alcohol-related**: history of excessive alcohol consumption; seizures occur during drinking bouts or immediately after withdrawal.
- **Others**: cardiac syncope, vasovagal episodes.

Differential diagnosis of confused behaviours occurring in the context of epilepsy

- **Post-ictal psychosis**: follows exacerbation of seizure activity; post-ictal latent period of normality before psychotic symptoms begin; clinical picture dominated by confusion, hallucinations, and affective disturbance (twilight state); history of previous episodes; usually lasts only a few days and is self-limiting.
- **Post-ictal confusion**: history of recent seizure; patient confused and drowsy; usually resolves within about 2 hours.
- **Alcohol intoxication**: evident signs of drunken behaviour; alcohol on breath; known history.
- **Head injury**: careful neurological examination indicated if recent history of head injury or evidence of scalp/facial injuries.
- **Anticonvulsant toxicity**: complaints of drowsiness, poor coordination; on examination nystagmus, dysarthria, and ataxia; there may be a history of recent change in drug dosage.

Immediate management
Related to epilepsy

1. If seizures are **well controlled**, find out from the patient who treated the epilepsy and where. Copy clinical correspondence with details of psychiatric diagnosis and treatment.
2. If seizures are **poorly controlled**, obtain details of medication, check compliance, request plasma anticonvulsant levels, and, once available, correspond as above.
3. The patient is **confused and disoriented**. This will usually be due to post-ictal confusion, but see previous differential diagnosis of confused behaviours. Post-ictal confusion will rarely exceed 6 hours. Observe until recovered; otherwise admit.
4. A **seizure** occurs. Most minor seizures are very brief and do not require any intervention. If a major tonic–clonic seizure occurs, ensure airway (turn patient on side and remove false teeth) and guard patient from hard-edged/cornered objects that could cause injury. Do not restrain or attempt to separate teeth. Give clonazepam 1–2 mg or Diazemuls®

10 mg intravenously. If the seizure is prolonged (>5 minutes) or status (repeated seizures without intervening recovery of consciousness) develops, repeat injection and request immediate medical assistance. Prolonged seizure activity/status is a medical emergency that may lead to hypoxia, hypotension, and hyperthermia, and may result in permanent brain damage.

Related to psychiatric illness

In general, immediate management is the same as it would be for the psychiatric condition if epilepsy were not present. However, there are exceptions.

- An **acute psychotic illness** in a patient not known to be psychotic is usually post-ictal. Unless relatives are used to dealing with such episodes, it is best to admit.
- **Non-epileptic seizures:** the clinician may suspect, and even observe, a seizure that appears non-epileptic. It is better to pass these observations on to the GP/specialist who usually treats a patient's epilepsy rather than comment directly. If in doubt, treat as for epilepsy.

Response to treatment

Commonly prescribed anticonvulsant drugs

- **Sodium valproate, carbamazepine,** and **lamotrigine** are first-choice anticonvulsants. Valproate is first-line for all seizure types. Carbamazepine is first-line only for focal epilepsy and is ineffective for absence and myoclonic seizures.
- **Levetiracetam** and **topiramate** are second-line drugs in generalized and focal epilepsy.
- **Phenytoin** and **phenobarbital** are effective but little used now due to long-term side-effects and risk in overdose.
- **Ethosuximide** is a first-choice drug against absence seizures.
- **Clonazepam, clobazam, gabapentin,** and **vigabatrin** are add-on therapies.

In women, pregnancy planning is essential because of the teratogenic risks of anticonvulsants. Folic acid reduces the risk of neural tube defects. N.B. carbamazepine reduces blood levels of oestrogen and progesterone and has implications for effective contraception.

Measuring blood drug levels is indicated to test compliance or toxicity (e.g. nausea, ataxia, confusion, diplopia). Blood levels do not correlate with therapeutic levels.

Some patients with intractable epilepsy may be eligible for brain surgery.

Course

In most patients (approximately 80 per cent), seizures will be effectively controlled by the first anticonvulsant prescribed. In patients with additional neurological and neuropsychiatric disabilities, control may not be so readily achieved and polytherapy may be unavoidable. Partial seizures are more difficult to control than primary generalized seizures.

Generalized absence seizures usually resolve by the third decade. Seizures developing for the first time in middle or late life may be associated with progressive underlying pathology and should be investigated with particular care.

Investigations

The investigation of newly suspected epileptic seizures includes FBC, ESR, U&Es, LFTs, calcium, glucose, EEG, and, particularly in the case of partial seizures, a search for a primary cause. This includes brain imaging (MRI) with specific views of the hippocampi if complex partial seizures. A waking scalp EEG will only show relevant abnormalities in about 50 per cent of cases; a sleep EEG is often more informative. In the case of epilepsy of late onset, periodic rescanning may be desirable.

When there is considerable doubt on clinical grounds about the epileptic nature of the seizures and the routine EEG remains negative, a prolonged EEG (telemetry)/video recording may capture a seizure and confirm or refute the diagnosis. In most centres, this investigation is carried out over a 5-day period whilst the patient is in hospital. Seizures must occur with sufficient frequency for this to be an effective investigation.

Patients considered for surgery may undergo tests that assist in localization. These may include telemetry with special electrode placement (foramen ovale, subdural, intracerebral), specialized MRI procedures, detailed neuropsychological assessment, and carotid amytal studies to determine cerebral dominance and lateralization of memory function.

Sexual and relationship problems

Sexual dysfunctions and desire disorders

The problems presenting in the male are:
- erectile disorder (impotence)
- premature ejaculation
- delayed ejaculation
- loss of desire.

The problems presenting in the female are:
- vaginismus (painful spasmodic contraction of the muscles surrounding the vagina, usually impeding intercourse; it may be caused by fear or aversion to coitus but can also have organic aetiology)
- orgasmic dysfunction
- dyspareunia (pain during intercourse)
- loss of desire.

Problems deriving from the relationship include:
- incompatibility of sexual desire
- conflict over sexual preferences and practices.

The history is best taken from both partners separately, at least in part, but much of it can be usefully obtained from a joint interview, which also affords the possibility of direct observation of the couple. An empathic, non-judgemental approach is needed.

Pointers in taking a sexual history are:
- Age at puberty (voice breaking, shaving, menarche).
- Age at which first ejaculation occurred.
- Age at first masturbation. How was this regarded? Fantasies? Anxieties?
- Attitudes of parents to sexual matters.
- Sexual seduction or childhood sexual abuse?

- Any unusual sexual preferences? Fantasies? Activities?
- Homosexual or heterosexual orientation (fantasies, desires, and experiences)?
- Any gender dysphoria, including non-arousing cross-dressing?
- Previous sexual experiences and relationships including painful or traumatic ones.
- Age at first intercourse.
- Current sex life (if any). Marital, extramarital, cohabiting?
- Current frequency of masturbation.
- Level of sexual drive. Any changes during this illness?
- Contraception? Safe sex? Sexually transmitted diseases?
- Sexual dysfunctions. Desire, arousal, or orgasm? Partner satisfied?
- Discrepancy in sexual interest between partners.
- Menopause? Hysterectomy? Hormone replacement?

Inquire into alcohol intake, smoking, spinal injuries, diabetes, hypertension, psychiatric illness and its medication, physical illness, surgical operations, stress, prior traumatic experiences (including sexual abuse or rape), recent life events, life-cycle stage, etc.

Obtain a picture of the **quality of general relationship**: communication, resentment, inhibitions, distance and closeness, invalidism, power, commitment. Any infidelities? Satisfaction with sexual life? Problems with fertility? Duration of present relationship? Sexual preferences and practices? Inhibitions?

Referral of the couple to a sexual disorder clinic is preferable, though dealing with the side-effects of drugs (e.g. antidepressants, antipsychotics) can sometimes obviate the need for referral. A **physical examination** is not always necessary. However, it is usually recommended in cases of erectile disorder and vaginismus, but should be conducted by a specialist (e.g. urologist or the patient's gynaecologist).

Sexual deviations and variations

They may vary greatly in severity and in relevance, from very minor activities in an ongoing relationship to harmful practices. Denial is a common phenomenon in those with extreme sexual deviations because of their conflict with societal values and norms. Examples of **harmful deviations** include paedophilia, zoophilia, necrophilia, public masturbation, voyeurism, obscene telephone calls, frotteurism (touching people sexually in crowds), stealing clothing (to use fetishistically), and the more dangerous forms of sadomasochism including sex murder.

The challenge at interview is to obtain a truthful account.

- Details of the **deviant behaviour**: how often, where, when, with whom, whether caught and/or convicted, whether fantasies are associated, etc. Ask about deviant behaviours other than the one presenting.
- What thoughts and feelings are experienced? What visual images or materials are used to achieve arousal? Does the person have a normal sexual outlet as well as the deviant one? What are the masturbatory fantasies?
- How high is the sexual drive (may be judged by masturbatory frequency or desired frequency of ejaculation)?

- How dangerous is the activity? Is it against the law? Does it damage the patient or others? Is there any empathy with possible victims?
- Do family members or partner know about the activities? What is their attitude?
- Past criminal history (related to this behaviour or others).
- Is the patient motivated by the wish to change his/her behaviour or simply to avoid punishment?
- Is there an associated sexual dysfunction in more 'normal' sexual activities?

Referral to forensic psychotherapy services may be appropriate in patients with potentially harmful sexual deviations. More severe deviations which have included rape or child sexual abuse should involve forensic psychiatric services following criminal conviction.

Gender identity disorder

It is important not to move too quickly into gender reassignment procedures, and it is usual to recommend that the patient should live as a member of the opposite sex for a period of 2 years, usually with the aid of hormone therapy, before any consideration of surgery. It is then possible to carry out gender reassignment operations, with hormone therapy, in selected cases, but a great deal of counselling is necessary after surgery and adjustment is variable.

Couple relationship therapy

Pointers in history taking are:
- number of previous engagements or serious relationships
- difficulties in these and reasons for breakup
- age at present marriage (or cohabitation); reasons (e.g. pregnancy)
- age, occupation, health, and personality of partner
- quality of relationship; threat of separation or divorce
- reaction of partner to patient's present illness
- communication, negotiation of differences, ability to confide, empathy
- dominance, submission, distance, trust, fidelity, jealousy
- problems (past and present), arguments, violence
- death of spouse, separation (temporary or permanent), divorce
- changes in sexual activities during relationship (e.g. ageing effects)
- obstetric history: pregnancies, live births, terminations, and miscarriages
- children (present or earlier relationships)
  - ages, gender, names
  - present and past health: sick child? Any psychiatric problems or treatment?
  - attitude towards children and future pregnancies
  - proximity and contact with children not now living at home.

Relationship problems are common both in themselves and in the context of many psychiatric difficulties. Couple therapy provides a framework, and the consent of both partners is required. In the couple interview, therapists will elicit details of the presenting problem, other strains in the relationship, the general satisfaction and commitment of both partners, the good aspects and troublesome aspects of the relationship, the risk of divorce or separation, problems with children, housing and financial problems, sexual satisfaction, and what attracted them to each other. Have there been major quarrels or violence? Infidelity? What are the resentments on both sides? Do they confide in each other? Who is more upset by the current problems? In couple therapy, like family therapy, no clear distinction is made between assessment and treatment. The first session aims to establish a treatment contract and this is reviewed regularly.

Treatments

Most of the sections in this chapter concern advice on early treatment. The medications relate to adults. Advice on rapid tranquillization for acute behavioural disturbances is given in Table 9.1.

Acute psychosis

First-episode patients

Ideally, patients should be treated by a specialized first-onset team. Patients should receive an antipsychotic chosen jointly by the prescriber and the properly informed patient or carer (or both). Although many psychiatrists believe that atypical or second-generation antipsychotics (SGAs) are superior to first-generation antipsychotics (FGAs), the CATIE and CUtLASS studies have weakened the basis for this belief. Indeed, meta-analyses show that there is little to choose between the majority of the available antipsychotics in effectiveness.

Therefore, the different profile of side-effects, once communicated to the patient and/or carer, should usually inform the choice of medication (see Appendix 5). Extrapyramidal side-effects (EPSEs) are common with use of the typical or first-generation antipsychotics (FGAs), whereas weight

Table 9.1 Acute disturbed or violent behaviour

Step	Actions	Additional considerations
1	Try non-drug measures: seclusion, talking down, privacy and quiet	
2	Offer oral lorazepam 1–2 mg. Repeat every 45–60 minutes. Go to step 3 if three doses fail.	Offer oral olanzapine 10 mg, or risperidone 1–2 mg, or haloperidol 5 mg, if not taking regular antipsychotic.
3	Consider IM treatment: lorazepam 1–2 mg, or olanzapine 10 mg, or aripiprazole 9.75 mg, or haloperidol 5 mg plus promethazine 50 mg. Promethazine 50 mg IM is an alternative in patients who are tolerant to benzodiazepines. Repeat at interval of 30–60 minutes if insufficient effect.	IM olanzapine should not be combined with IM benzodiazepines. Haloperidol not first line due to dystonic risk and pre-treatment ECG recommendations. IM/IV procliclidine 5–10 mg should be to hand in case of acute dystonia.
4	Consider IV treatment. Diazepam 10 mg over at least 5 minutes.	Repeat after 5–10 minutes if insufficient effects (up to three times). IV flumazenil 200 mcg should be to hand in case of respiratory depression.
5	Seek expert advice. Amobarbital 250 mg IM is an option.	Very, very few episodes of rapid tranquillization should reach this point.

gain, dyslipidaemia, and, ultimately, diabetes or metabolic syndrome can result from atypical or second-generation antipsychotics (SGAs). Other troublesome antipsychotic side-effects include sedation, postural hypotension, elevated prolactin, sexual dysfunction, seizures, and prolonged QT interval.

Appendices 5, 6, and 7 contain further information about antipsychotics. Information about management of the side-effects of clozapine is given in Appendix 7.

Initially, a single antipsychotic should be used at its minimum effective dose for a period of 2 weeks before any increment is attempted. This is with the exception of depot medication, where assessment of efficacy or change of dose needs to take into account a longer time frame (see following details). If the drug is not effective or cannot be tolerated, a second agent should be substituted for a similar period of time and titrated accordingly until clinical response is obtained. If there is no response to the second antipsychotic (FGA or SGA), clozapine should then be used as it is superior for the care of those who have failed to respond to adequate doses of two other antipsychotics; in most countries, its use is confined to these treatment-resistant patients because of its side-effects (see Appendix 7).

Subsequent episodes

Relapses in people with schizophrenia and other serious psychotic disorders are commonly due to stress or non-adherence. Understanding adherence is best approached within the context of a continuing relationship with the patient. If non-adherence is due to poor tolerability of the medication, then a different agent should be offered, but if it is driven by non-medical beliefs about illness, denial, lack of awareness of illness, or other factors such as illicit drug use, disorganized life style, or poor support, then a broader approach will need to be taken. Depot medication can be useful for patients who do not take oral medications reliably. In such cases, patients should be presented with all the available options, as some might experience injectable antipsychotics as coercive, whilst others might prefer it to the commitment of taking tablets daily. Following initiating depot medication, plasma levels continue to increase for 6–12 weeks from the first dose. Therefore, any assessment of efficacy or change of dose needs to take into account this longer time frame.

Non-pharmacological treatment

It is essential that the pharmacological treatments mentioned should be combined with attempts to resolve any obvious precipitating factors. Cognitive behavioural therapy should be available for all who are willing and able to accept it. If the patient's psychosis persists, the possibility of underlying mood disorder should be considered and an antidepressant or mood stabilizer introduced where appropriate.

Important side-effects of antipsychotic medication and their treatment

Acute dystonia

Abrupt onset of muscle spasm hours after commencing an antipsychotic (particularly a FGA) can be very alarming and, naturally, may adversely affect future adherence. It is more common in the young, especially on first exposure to antipsychotics. If it causes respiratory stridor, oculogyric crisis, or tongue protrusion, it can induce panic. If it is suspected, one should give procyclidine 5–10 mg IM or IV and stop the antipsychotic. Be quick to check for cyanosis, give oxygen, and transfer to a medical unit or to the nearest A&E department as required. Monitor for changes in oxygen saturation, pulse, and blood pressure.

Neuroleptic malignant syndrome

Neuroleptic malignant syndrome (NMS) is a rare and idiosyncratic sympathetic hyperactivity reaction to dopaminergic antagonism characterized by rigidity and other dystonias, fever, autonomic dysfunction (fluctuating blood pressure, tachycardia), diaphoresis, and clouding of consciousness. There is substantial overlap with acute lethal catatonia. The incidence of the condition is variously reported as between 0.07 and 2 per cent, probably because of the lack of clear diagnostic criteria and the overlap with other severe extrapyramidal syndromes. Associated biochemical and other abnormalities include a grossly elevated creatine kinase, leucocytosis, abnormal LFTs, and raised erythrocyte sedimentation rate.

NMS has been reported with all antipsychotics but also, occasionally, with antidepressants and lithium. It tends to be associated with larger doses of high-potency antipsychotics (FGAs mainly), recent or rapid dose change (increase or reduction), hyperthyroidism, dehydration, and agitation. Reported mortality varies between 12 and 18 per cent, usually as a consequence of autonomic instability (e.g. cardiac arrest) or renal failure due to rhabdomyolysis and myoglobinuria. The mortality may be lower with SGAs.

Treatment of neuroleptic malignant syndrome

This is a life-threatening condition, so when the diagnosis of NMS is suspected, antipsychotic medication should be stopped immediately and vital signs monitored. If the diagnosis is confirmed or strongly suspected, the patient should be transferred to a medical intensive care facility (see Table 9.2). Withdrawal of antipsychotic medication usually produces rapid resolution of symptoms in patients identified early. In the medical unit, full supportive measures to maintain hydration electrolyte status and renal and respiratory function should be available. A dopamine agonist such as oral bromocriptine, in combination with dantrolene to relax peripheral muscles, can be useful. Sedation should be administered with benzodiazepines. In established cases, these measures should lead to a resolution over about 10 days.

A 'drug holiday' of at least 5 days, and preferably longer, while the symptoms and signs of NMS resolve completely, is recommended and diminishes the chance of recurrence on re-challenge. Consult an expert

Table 9.2 Algorithm for the treatment of neuroleptic malignant syndrome

Transfer to acute medical ward or intensive care unit
Monitor ECG, blood pressure, and renal status
↓
Cessation of neuroleptics
↓
Bromocriptine 5–10 mg orally three times daily
↓
(if unable to swallow)
Apomorphine infusion 1 mg/h sc
↓
(no response)
Dantrolene sodium 50 mg twice daily maximum for 3 days

in psychopharmacology before re-challenge. About one in six patients will suffer a recurrence after a re-challenge.

Mania and hypomania

Acute mania or hypomania usually requires pharmacological treatment to reduce harm. If mania or hypomania occurs whilst a patient is taking anti-depressant medication, the first step should be to stop any antidepressant treatment before initiating antimanic treatment.

The first episode of mania or hypomania is best treated with:
1. An antipsychotic in case of disturbed, chaotic, or agitated behaviour. Options are:
    a. Olanzapine (10 mg/day increasing to 20 mg/day if needed)
    b. Aripiprazole (15 mg/day increasing to 30 mg/day)
    c. Risperidone (3 mg/day increasing to 6 mg/day)
    d. Quetiapine XL (300 mg/day 1 and 600 mg/day 2)
    e. Haloperidol (5–10 mg/day increasing to 15 mg/day).
2. Sodium valproate (as semi-sodium 250 mg TDS or as sodium valproate slow release 500 mg/day, increased according to tolerability and target plasma concentrations (trough (predose)) of 125 mg/l or to 30 mg/ kg/day). Not recommended in women of child-bearing potential.
3. Lithium (at a dose of 400 mg daily, increasing 200 mg every 4 days until target plasma concentrations (measured as 12 hours post-dose) reach 0.4–0.75 mmol/l). Requires long-term adherence with monitoring to prevent acute toxicity that reliably occurs at levels >1.5 mmol/l with severe GI and CNS symptoms.

The doses of these drugs should not be escalated simply to achieve a seda-tive effect.

If the behavioural disturbance requires sedation, one may initiate benzo-diazepine (lorazepam or clonazepam up to 4 mg/day) but should remember to withdraw it after resolution of the acute symptoms.

In severely disturbed patients refusing medication, parenteral treatment with benzodiazepine may be useful (diazemuls 10 mg IV over 5 mins and repeated after 5–10 mins if insufficient, up to 3 times) but requires both an emergency team and flumazenil to hand.

Electroconvulsive therapy (ECT) may very occasionally be considered. This should be bilateral because of the need for a rapid response. The disturbance usually abates after the first few sessions.

Catatonia

Catatonia is a severe movement disorder characterized by immobility or waxy flexibility, negativism, automatic obedience, mutism, echolalia, echopraxia, and a 'wooden' affect; rarely, this may switch into excessive purpose-less activity. If these symptoms are accompanied by autonomic instability or hyperthermia, a diagnosis of malignant catatonia is made, which is impossible to distinguish from NMS.

Treatment of the catatonia is of the underlying condition, but in persistent or distressing states or where dehydration, pulmonary embolism, or aspiration are potential harms, benzodiazepines or even ECT may be tried. Benzodiazepines are the first-line treatment and the majority of patients respond to standard doses of lorazepam (up to 4 mg/day) although, in some cases, higher doses, with monitoring, may be needed.

Severe depression

Antidepressant treatment

Milder forms of depression can be treated with psychological interventions such as cognitive–behavioural therapy (CBT) or interpersonal therapy (IPT), as outlined in NICE guidance. Antidepressants are recommended in cases of moderate to severe depression and can be administered in combination with high-intensity psychological intervention such as CBT or IPT.

An antidepressant should be chosen from the SSRI class (e.g. fluoxetine, sertraline) after an initial discussion with the patient regarding desired outcome and delayed therapeutic effect, side-effects, and discontinuation effects. Once the antidepressant has been selected, the medication should be prescribed according to BNF recommendations and the therapeutic effect of the treatment should be assessed over a 2-week period. If a partial response is observed, treatment should be maintained for a period of up to 9 months, or for 6 months after the resolution of symptoms, unless the patient has had two prior episodes of depression and functional impairment, in which case, antidepressant treatment can be recommended for 2 years.

Patients should be monitored during the initial stages of treatment for the appearance of restlessness, agitation, and suicidality, as well as for agent-specific side-effects (such as gastrointestinal disturbances, anorexia and weight loss, hypersensitivity reactions, sexual dysfunction, arthralgia, myalgia, and photosensitivity). If the medication is poorly tolerated, a different antidepressant should be used.

If no response is observed after the first 2 weeks and side-effects are negligible, the dose should be increased and the response monitored over a further 2 weeks. If after 3–4 weeks, no therapeutic effect has been observed, a different antidepressant should be used.

When switching between antidepressants, abrupt withdrawal should be avoided and cross-tapering should be used. All antidepressants (but especially paroxetine and venlafaxine) have the potential to cause discontinuation phenomena when stopped. Common symptoms of antidepressant discontinuation are dizziness, electric shock sensations, anxiety and agitation, insomnia, influenza-like symptoms, diarrhoea and abdominal spasms, paraesthesia, mood swings, nausea, and low mood. If withdrawal symptoms occur, return to the last dose tolerated by the patient, and then slow the subsequent rate of drug withdrawal. If the drug has been stopped, give reassurance; symptoms rarely last more than 1–2 weeks.

If the patient does not respond to a second antidepressant, check adherence and review the formulation; consider personality, alcohol use, and social factors which may be aggravating the patient's condition. An antidepressant from a different class may be tried e.g. tricyclic (TCA). Alternatively, an atypical antipsychotic may be added if the depression is severe, especially if there are psychotic symptoms.

'Treatment-resistant' depression is usually defined as failure to respond to adequate trials of two antidepressants or one antidepressant and ECT. The following strategies could be used:

1. First line:
   a. Add lithium, if compliance is good and patient agrees to monitoring. Therapeutic range for treatment-resistant depression in the short term is higher than that for mania at 0.4–1.0 mmol/l. Nevertheless, it is important to closely monitor kidney function as chronic lithium levels >0.8 mmol/l are associated with greater risk of renal toxicity.
   b. Add liothyronine sodium (T3) (20–50 micrograms/day) under thyroid function monitoring.
   c. Add bupropion (up to 400 mg/day) to an SSRI.
   d. Add an atypical antipsychotic (quetiapine up to 300 mg/day, risperidone up to 3 mg/day, and aripiprazole up to 20 mg/day) to an SSRI.
   e. Combine olanzapine (12.5 mg/day) with fluoxetine (50 mg/day).
   f. Combine an SSRI or venlafaxine with mianserin (up to 30 mg/day) or with mirtazapine (up to 45 mg/day).
   g. Consider ECT for severe life-threatening depression when a rapid response is needed.
2. Second line:
   a. Venlafaxine (at doses higher than 200 mg/day) with BP monitoring.
   b. Add lamotrigine (up to 400 mg/day).
   c. Add buspirone (up to 60 mg/day) to an SSRI.
   d. Add pindolol (5 mg TDS or 7.5 mg OD).

For psychotic depression, TCAs are first line, unless they are poorly tolerated, in which case SSRIs/SNRIs are preferred. Olanzapine (up to

20 mg/day) or quetiapine (up to 750 mg/day) can be used as augmentation strategy. Quetiapine is licensed for use as an adjunctive therapy in major depressive disorder.

Eventually, following resolution of symptoms, the antidepressant should be withdrawn gradually and the patient should be informed of discontinuation effects he/she may experience.

Prescribing during pregnancy and breastfeeding

General principles

Clinicians should discuss the possibility of pregnancy with any woman of child-bearing age who is receiving, or will receive, medication for a mental disorder. The discussion should help the individual understand and manage medication risks and should be well documented. Try to involve the woman in the decision about her medication plan as much as possible, in order for her to have a sense of agency over her care and, indirectly, that of her unborn child.

Topics to discuss should include GP support with contraception, folic acid supplements, severity of symptoms and frequency of relapses, effect of the untreated symptoms or disorder on the patient and also on a fetus, the effect of medication on symptoms and on a fetus. Occasionally, child protection procedures and potential involvement of social services following delivery will require discussion.

Try to keep in mind the woman's medication history. Unless a medication is explicitly contraindicated, it may be better to prescribe something that has been effective in the past, even though it is not a first-line agent in perinatal cases. This may contribute to a speedier recovery, avoid polypharmacy, as well as contribute to better adherence.

It is important not to interrupt a medication plan abruptly if a patient discovers she is pregnant. Abrupt discontinuation of medication during pregnancy leads to relapse in many cases. If a woman states she is pregnant, it would be best to make a plan with her concerning her medication, replacing more teratogenic agents with less harmful ones where possible and, if needed, seeking the advice of perinatal psychiatrists or pharmacists.

Patients should be referred to the local perinatal team or, in its absence, be managed in close liaison with the local obstetrics team. Monotherapy should be sought whenever possible and the drug with the lowest risk to mother and fetus should be used at its lowest effective dose, with close monitoring of plasma drug levels, mental state, and fetal development. Elective Cesarean sections have the advantage of a degree of planning and control and may be recommended in some cases. Following birth, the neonate should be kept under close observation and screened for signs of drug withdrawal.

Antipsychotics

Patients with established psychotic disorders who are being treated with antipsychotic medication should be advised to remain on medication during pregnancy.

FGAs (chlorpromazine, haloperidol and trifluoperazine) are lowest risk in pregnancy and are the treatment of choice in most cases if their side-effects can be tolerated. Depot medication and anticholinergics are best avoided during pregnancy, according to current NICE guidance.

Regarding SGAs, the agents with most data accrued to date are clozapine and olanzapine. Both are associated with gestational diabetes. Clozapine has been associated with neonatal seizures, so olanzapine is currently considered to be the safest SGA.

Antidepressants

Antidepressant medication is recommended for moderate to severe depressive illness and for those who develop the disorder during pregnancy.

Older agents such as tricyclic antidepressants have been extensively studied during pregnancy and are considered lowest risk. Their antimuscarinic side-effects (dry mouth, dry nose, blurred vision, constipation, and sedation) may be troublesome to pregnant women and, as a class, are generally thought to increase the risk of preterm delivery. Furthermore, they can be more dangerous in overdose and, therefore, should be avoided in those thought at high risk of suicide. Among tricyclics, amitriptyline and imipramine are recommended.

The newer and easier tolerated SSRIs are also accruing safety data during pregnancy. Sertraline is currently first-choice treatment due to extensive data mostly indicating no teratogenic effect, despite being associated with an increased risk of earlier delivery and reduced birthweight. Paroxetine is not recommended as it appears to be associated with cardiac malformations if used at doses higher than 25 mg/day during the first trimester of pregnancy.

MAOIs are best avoided during pregnancy because of their heightened risk for congenital malformations and association with hypertension in pregnant women.

Mood stabilizers

Anticonvulsants and lithium should generally be considered unsafe in pregnancy and their use is discouraged because of teratogenicity.

Patients needing mood stabilizing agents, due to bipolar affective disorder, should be made aware that either a medication-free period during the first trimester or treatment with antipsychotic medication are recommended.

A drug-free trial is only advisable if the symptoms are mild to moderate and their onset gradual rather than abrupt, there is no past history of DSH, suicide, vulnerability, or violence against others when unwell, and the patient has good insight, a supportive social network, and quick access to services. There should be access to a hospital specialist service (such as Mother and Baby Unit).

Pointers to continuing medication would include: a high risk of relapse, inability to monitor the patient safely off medication (in the community or in hospital), severe symptoms with abrupt onset, a past history of serious self-harm, vulnerability or aggression towards others when unwell. Reasons should be discussed and explored with the patient and clearly stated in the patient's notes.

Women remaining on lithium should undergo level 2 ultrasound screening for Ebstein's anomaly at 6 and 18 weeks.

For acute manic episodes during pregnancy, an antipsychotic is the first-line treatment, followed by ECT if there is no observable improvement. For depressive episodes during pregnancy, CBT should be used for mild to moderate episodes and an SSRI for more severe cases of depression.

Rapid tranquillization

Pregnant women requiring emergency management of acutely disturbed behaviour should receive treatment with antihistamines such as promethazine or short-acting benzodiazepines such as lorazepam. In cases in which the behavioural disturbance is thought to be secondary to psychosis, an antipsychotic could also be used, and some Mother and Baby Units prefer using FGAs for sedation and rapid tranquillization.

Breast-feeding

Psychotropic medications pass into breast milk. The risks and benefits of breast-feeding should be discussed with the mother. Benefits of breast-feeding for the baby include an enhanced immunological response and resistance to infections, a reduced incidence of gastrointestinal disturbances, a reduced risk of obesity as an adult, and a reduced risk of developing eczema. The benefits for the mother include cost, convenience, and sterility (compared to bottle-feeding), and reduced risk of developing ovarian cancer. Breast-feeding often helps create a strong emotional bond between mother and baby.

Medication should always be prescribed as monotherapy, administered at the lowest effective dose within BNF limits and, whenever possible, feeding should take place when maternal plasma drug levels are not at their peak.

If an *antidepressant* is needed, sertraline is the drug of choice as infant serum levels appear to be low and no adverse effects have been noted in the children of mothers treated with it.

If an *antipsychotic* is needed, sulpiride or olanzapine should be the first choice, but others such as haloperidol, chlorpromazine, quetiapine, and risperidone can also be used with enhanced monitoring of the baby's development. The use of clozapine is discouraged by NICE because of its risk of neutropenia and seizures.

Mood stabilizers are not advised in breast-feeding. Lithium treatment in the mother has been associated with adverse effects in the baby and NICE advises against its use. If valproate is used, contraceptive measures need to be put in place, and valproate carries a risk of hepatotoxicity in the breast-fed infant. Lamotrigine carries a risk of rash in the infant and it is not recommended in breast-feeding. If a mood stabilizer is needed, and the mother wishes to breast-feed, an antipsychotic with mood-stabilizing properties is preferable.

For *sedation*, antihistamines such as promethazine or a short-acting benzodiazepine such as lorazepam can be used. Zolpidem can be used for *night sedation*. Mothers should be advised not to sleep next to their babies whilst taking sedatives.

Electroconvulsive therapy (ECT)

ECT is probably the most effective treatment available for severe depression but is now used much less frequently than formerly. It involves seizure induction and is associated with cognitive side-effects (e.g. mild retrograde amnesia).

Indications

NICE has issued guidance on ECT. Currently, it recommends ECT be restricted to severe depressive illness, a prolonged or severe episode of mania, or catatonia, where the clinical situation is life-threatening or requires a fast improvement of severe symptoms.

The number of treatments given during a course of ECT ranges between six and twelve, and they are given twice a week. Clinical response and monitoring should be ongoing as some patients respond with less than six treatments. In rare cases, fortnightly or monthly treatment is prescribed as maintenance therapy or relapse prevention strategy.

NICE does not recommend the use of ECT for prevention of recurrence of depressive illness, or for the general management of schizophrenia.

Patients and relatives are generally wary of ECT and great care should be taken in explaining the procedure, treatment aims, and side-effects, both general and specific, to the individual. Information leaflets to help people to make an informed decision about their treatment should be made available in formats and languages that will make them accessible to a wide range of service users.

Mental health law regulating ECT is outlined in Chapter 10, 'A note on ECT', p. 164. Every doctor should make himself familiar with the local policy for ECT.

Detailed information about ECT can be found in the most recent third edition of the *The ECT Handbook* (Royal College of Psychiatrists, 2013). This, as well as information for the general public, can be downloaded from the Royal College of Psychiatrists website: <http://www.rcpsych.ac.uk/usefulresources/publications.aspx>.

Depressive illnesses

ECT is a proven effective treatment for depression and should not be considered a last resort option. It can also be safely administered to patients with physical illnesses, the elderly, and during pregnancy.

ECT in depression is recommended as a *first-line treatment* for:
1. the emergency treatment of depression where a rapid definitive response is needed
2. patients with high suicidal risk
3. patients with severe psychomotor retardation and associated problems of eating and drinking or physical deterioration
4. patients who suffer from treatment-resistant depression and who have responded to ECT in previous episodes of illness
5. patients who are pregnant, if there is concern about the teratogenic effects of antidepressants and antipsychotics
6. patients for whom it is the preferred choice of treatment and for whom there are strong clinical indications for its use.

ECT is *second-line treatment* for:
1. patients with treatment-resistant depression
2. patients who experience severe side-effects from medication, limiting effective treatment
3. patients whose medical or psychiatric condition, in spite of adequate pharmacotherapy, has deteriorated to an extent that raises concern.

Old-age psychiatrists may recommend its use in the depressed elderly who have not responded to drug treatments or have suffered unpleasant side-effects. Remission rates in clinical trials are 60–70 per cent.

Manic illness
ECT may be considered for severe mania associated with life-threatening physical exhaustion or treatment resistance. Indications include the need for a speedy therapeutic response, as a safe alternative to high-dose medications, or if patients have drug-resistant or 'rapid cycling' mania.

Schizophrenia
There are very few indications for ECT in schizophrenia. Very rarely, it may be used when psychotic symptoms are associated with abnormal motor activity such as catatonic excitement or immobility. It may be considered if the patient cannot tolerate medications or has failed to respond to adequate doses of antipsychotics including clozapine. However, even if there is short-term benefit, after this treatment one must rely on more conventional approaches.

Catatonia
ECT may be considered as a first-line treatment in life-threatening malignant catatonia when treatment with lorazepam has been ineffective.

Contraindications
Although there are no absolute contraindications to ECT, coexisting medical illnesses must be treated. Close liaison between the psychiatrist, anaesthetist, and physicians is necessary. Pregnancy and old age are not contraindications to ECT, but any contraindications to general anaesthesia will apply; 'high-risk' cases with recent myocardial infarction, cerebrovascular accident, or raised intracranial pressure should be assessed on an individual basis in consultation with the anaesthetist. Those with known cardiac disease will need assessment by a physician or cardiologist prior to ECT. ECG monitoring is necessary during ECT administration, and staff should be adequately trained in cardiopulmonary resuscitation and management of arrhythmias. Following myocardial infarction or stroke, ECT should be delayed as long as possible and is probably safer after 3 months.

Complications
The principal adverse outcomes of ECT are mortality and cognitive adverse effects.

The mortality associated with ECT is similar to that for minor surgical procedures (estimated to be 1 per 10,000 patients or 1 per 80,000 treatments).

Anterograde amnesia is usually temporary but defects in retrograde memory, particularly for events closest to the time of treatment, can be more long-lasting. Autobiographical memory may be particularly affected with patients being distressed by failure to remember important events in their life. While bilateral application of ECT is currently the most common means of inducing a seizure, right unilateral ECT can be used if cognitive side-effects are troublesome but is less effective.

Other common post-ictal side-effects include headache and delirium. Rarer side-effects include asystole, apnoea, prolonged seizures, and physical complications such as ruptured bladder or aspiration pneumonia.

Preparation

Pretreatment evaluation should include:

1. a thorough physical examination, including an ECG, and appropriate blood tests (FBC, U&Es, and TFTs); CXR, EEG, and neuroimaging are not required unless indicated clinically
2. a history of personal and family responses to anesthesia
3. a dental examination
4. a thorough psychiatric evaluation including response to previous treatments
5. a cognitive assessment 2 days before and after.

The anaesthetist should be notified of any significant physical illnesses and current medication. As benzodiazepines are powerful anticonvulsants, they should be avoided prior to ECT unless there is a benzodiazepine dependence. Similarly, anticonvulsants raise the seizure threshold and so higher stimulus energies may be needed for treatment. Anticonvulsants prescribed for mood stabilization may be continued during ECT. Antipsychotics tend to be proconvulsant and they can be prescribed the night before the treatment with the knowledge and consent of the anaesthetist.

In preparation for *anaesthesia*, patients should be fasted for at least 6 hours before the procedure to ensure there are no gastric contents that could be regurgitated and cause aspiration during the recovery.

All patients should be accompanied to the ECT suite by a named nurse or a member of staff well known to them. Staff should have completed a pre-ECT checklist, detailing general observations including removal of jewellery and dentures as appropriate. The consultant's signed prescription for ECT and documents detailing the psychiatric and medical history and the medications should also be available. If the patient has had ECT before, previous prescription charts can give useful information about the stimulus charge required and should be made available. Fully informed consent must be obtained and documented, or the relevant legal documents pertinent to the administration of ECT must be available for scrutiny.

Administration

Prior to anaesthesia, administration of anticholinergics (atropine, glycopyrronium bromide) reduces the risk of post-ictal bradycardia. In addition, they minimize the risk of aspiration by reducing oral and respiratory secretions. Neuromuscular blockers (suxamethonium) are administered prior to electric stimulation to prevent bone fractures and physical injury related to convulsions.

The team usually consists of a consultant psychiatrist, a consultant anaesthetist, a psychiatric nurse, and a general nurse with specialist training in intensive care. The doctor administering the ECT would always be the psychiatrist, and he should either be a consultant or being supervised by one and be familiar with the ECT machine.

Most modern machines deliver brief pulses and have an EEG monitoring facility. The EEG is now the definitive method for measuring seizure duration and can also provide useful information about seizure quality. Prolonged seizures are those that last for 2 minutes or more and should be terminated either with further induction agent or intravenous diazepam.

Electrode placement can be either bilateral or right unilateral. Bilateral placement is currently more routinely used and may be preferable where a rapid response is required, but unilateral placement is associated with less memory impairment and regaining orientation more quickly.

In the bifrontotemporal position (or bilateral), electrodes are placed at each side of the frontotemporal region with the centre of each electrode approximately 4 cm above the midpoint of an imaginary line drawn from the external auditory meatus (tragus) to the lateral angle of the eye (lateral canthus).

In the right unilateral position, one electrode is typically placed in the aforementioned position and the other is placed on the centroparietal scalp, lateral to the midline vertex. As the left hemisphere is dominant in most people, unilateral electrode placement is almost always over the right hemisphere.

Using a method called *empirical titration* during the first session, progressively higher doses of charge are given until the seizure threshold is established. This is the stimulus charge required to induce a seizure lasting more than 15 seconds in motor activity or 25 seconds on EEG monitoring. The first stimulation at the first treatment a patient receives is usually 25–50 mC. Once the threshold is established, the initial electrical dose should be at least 50 per cent above it and 50–100 per cent above where emergency treatment is required to save life. If clinical improvement is suboptimal after 4–6 treatments, the dose should be increased to 150 per cent above seizure threshold.

The *number of treatments* will be determined by the clinical progress, which should be formally documented in case notes. A common policy is twice weekly administration for 6–12 treatments.

Alcohol and drug misuse

The treatment of substance misuse is guided by two fundamental principles:
- First, obtain a good drug history to determine whether the pattern of substance use constitutes:
  - harmful use
  - dependent use (compulsion to use/craving, salience of drug use, narrowing of repertoire, increased (or decreased) tolerance, continued use despite harm, withdrawal symptoms, and reinstatement after abstinence)
  - polysubstance misuse.

- Secondly, conduct a good physical examination; polysubstance misuse is associated with multiple physical complications (see Chapter 8, 'Alcohol and drug use', p. 107).

Harm reduction

Many drug users who seek help will not see abstinence as a desirable or achievable goal; insisting on this from the first contact may result in the perception that they cannot be helped, or that the service cannot meet their needs, and discourage further help seeking. The spread of blood-borne viruses including HIV, among injecting drug users, prompted a re-evaluation of treatment services, leading to a pragmatic approach with the aim of reducing blood-borne virus spread, drug-related crime, preventing progression to injecting use, and engaging people in initial treatment.

A hierarchy of achievable intermediate treatment goals are agreed with the patient, for example, to reduce intravenous drug use and transfer to oral drug use, or to move from risky injecting where needles are being shared to safer injecting using clean injecting equipment. Basic harm reduction services should be available whenever a drug user presents to a service and should include the following:

- Advice on safe injecting techniques, including not sharing or reusing needles, skin cleaning, and advice about the danger of some injecting sites, particularly groin and femoral.
- Availability of sterile injecting equipment. This may be from a local drugs agency or a pharmacy needle-exchange scheme.
- Education on virus transmission and the correct use of condoms; free condoms.
- Advice about overdose risk, including awareness of losing tolerance after abstinence or lower drug intake, such as being in prison, the dangers of new supplies of drug which may have higher purity, and basic life support and help-seeking methods in the event of encountering overdose in another drug user.
- Advice on the dangers of prescribed and non-prescribed drugs to children.
- Hepatitis B immunization; HIV and hepatitis testing, with appropriate counselling.
- Access to appropriate psychosocial support services e.g. housing, legal and financial advice, counselling, medical and psychological support for sex workers.

Substitute opioid prescribing has the aim of eliminating illicit drug use but often reduces it rather than completely replaces it. It is effective in reducing blood-borne virus transmission and criminal activity, and helps people engage in initial stages of treatment and progress to longer-term treatment goals. There is no evidence to support substitute prescribing of stimulants or benzodiazepines.

Psychosocial interventions

Although attention to medical and psychiatric issues is crucial, psychosocial interventions form the cornerstone of alcohol and drug treatment in the form of flexible key working, self-help groups, and more formal group or individual interventions. Key working includes advice, harm reduction, therapeutic engagement, helping with social problems, and motivational interviewing. More formal psychosocial interventions include relapse prevention programmes. These can be delivered to individuals or groups and combine education, self-reflection, and practical advice for managing high-risk situations. Self-help groups such as Alcoholics Anonymous, Narcotics Anonymous, and SMART Recovery are effective and should be recommended to all patients. Family/couple therapy can be helpful. The presence or history of drug or alcohol problems is not in itself sufficient reason to deny a patient access to psychological treatment, though careful consideration needs to be given to whether psychiatric symptoms result from, or are comorbid with, drug or alcohol use.

Further reading

Miller, W.R. and Rollnick, S. (2013). *Motivational Interviewing: Helping People Change. 3rd Edition.* The Guildford Press, New York/London.

Strang, J. *et al.* (2012). *Medications in Recovery.* (UK) NHS; National Treatment Agency for Substance Misuse.

Alcohol dependence

The alcohol withdrawal syndrome

Individuals will only experience symptoms of alcohol withdrawal if they are physically dependent on it. Thus, some heavy drinkers experience no withdrawal symptoms, whereas others show evidence of mild or moderate withdrawal, and a few will develop a life-threatening disturbance.

Symptoms of alcohol withdrawal start approximately 3–6 hours after the last drink. Early symptoms include tremor, sweats, nausea, insomnia, and anxiety. Transient auditory hallucinations in clear consciousness may occur. There is a risk of alcohol withdrawal (generalized) seizures of between 10 and 60 hours; risk factors include hypoglycaemia, hypokalaemia, hypomagnesaemia, and concurrent epilepsy. Most alcohol withdrawal syndromes resolve within 72 hours of drinking cessation. The more severe the withdrawal, the longer the duration. All patients are at risk of Wernicke's encephalopathy, particularly if they have poor nutritional status. A few patients develop delirium tremens (DTs) around 72 hours after the last drink (as described in the following section). DTs and Wernicke's encephalopathy are medical emergencies requiring immediate hospital admission.

Treatment of acute alcohol withdrawal

Patients with alcohol dependence should receive inpatient or outpatient detoxification as a component of a comprehensive treatment programme including preparatory psychosocial work and arrangements for appropriate after-care. With appropriate daily monitoring, many patients can be detoxified safely and effectively in the community by a specialist addiction service. Large doses of multiple days of chlordiazepoxide should not be given to take away. Medical detoxification alone is associated with a high relapse rate; encountering a patient with mild signs of alcohol withdrawal is not an indication for immediate detoxification. Indications for immediate (unplanned) detoxification include:

- DTs
- Wernicke's encephalopathy
- Established alcohol withdrawal with high risk of DTs or seizures
- To facilitate necessary hospital admission for another medical or psychiatric condition.

In the inpatient setting, chlordiazepoxide is prescribed according to a symptom-triggered flexible regime over the first 24–48 hours, with dosage titrated against the severity of withdrawal symptoms. The CIWA scoring system for alcohol withdrawal symptoms is given in Appendix 4. There needs to be monitoring for both under and over sedation. The presence of alcohol dependence and severity of current withdrawal syndromes should be established by taking a history and examining, with the assistance of an alcohol withdrawal severity scale. The initial dose should be given with caution, in case the patient has recently ingested alcohol which is still being absorbed. This can be assessed clinically by serial examination for severity of withdrawal symptoms or serial breathalyzer readings. The patient should be reassessed every 2–4 hours and further doses of chlordiazepoxide given as required; once initial dosing has begun, the aim should be, as far as possible, to suppress all withdrawal symptoms. In patients with severe liver disease, a short-acting benzodiazepine such as oxazepam or lorazepam may be used. These have a lower risk of accumulation and toxicity. In patients taking opioids, benzodiazepines should be prescribed cautiously, by an experienced doctor, and with closer monitoring, as the combination can be lethal.

If the patient is still symptomatic after 24 hours, higher doses of chlordiazepoxide may be needed. Otherwise, the total 24-hour dose should be calculated and prescribed in four divided doses for the second day, and then reduced by 20 per cent a day over the following 5 days. If the patient develops seizures, DTs, or the emergence of significant withdrawal symptoms, then the dose of chlordiazepoxide should be reviewed; it is usually sufficient to return to the previous day's dose, then continue reduction at a slightly slower rate.

Appropriate treatment as described here should prevent the development of alcohol withdrawal seizures, and anticonvulsants are not routinely indicated.

Because of the risk of Wernicke's encephalopathy, prophylactic thiamine (vitamin B) supplementation must be given. The absorption of oral thiamine is poor and so one pair IM/IV ampoules of high-potency B-complex vitamins (Pabrinex®) should be given daily for 3–5 days (or thiamine 200–300 mg IM daily if Pabrinex® is unavailable). There is a rare risk of anaphylaxis and so suitable resuscitation facilities should be available.

The approach to symptom-triggered inpatient alcohol withdrawal treatment should be as follows:

- First 24 hours—no fixed doses. Chlordiazepoxide (20–40 mg prn) and thiamine (200–300 mg IM/IV) prescribed. Review patient every 2–4 hours, giving chlordiazepoxide to minimize withdrawal symptoms.
- Day 2—calculate the stabilized daily dose and the dosing regime for the detox (see worked example in Table 9.3).
- Day 3 onwards—total dose is reduced by ~20 per cent each day until no longer required (Table 9.3).

Table 9.3 Writing the prescription chart: a worked example

Day	Chlordiazepoxide dose/times				Total daily dose
	08:00	14:00	18:00	22:00	
1	40 mg @ 11:00, 20 mg @ 14:00, none needed @ 16:00, 40 mg @ 18:00, none needed @ 20:00, 20 mg @ 22:00, patient slept, 40 mg @ 04:00, patient slept, 20 mg @ 08:00				Total of 180 mg given over 24h from 11:00 on day 1 to 11:00 on day 2—this is the stabilized daily dose.
2	N/A	40 mg	40 mg	40 mg	60 mg has already been given after the last dose time on day 1, so the dose for the rest of day 2 is 180 mg – 60 mg = 120 mg, given in divided doses.
3	35 mg	35 mg	35 mg	40 mg	20% of 180 mg is ~35 mg, which is the daily dose reduction for rest of detox. 180 mg – 35 mg = 145 mg
4	30 mg	25 mg	25 mg	30 mg	110 mg
5	20 mg	15 mg	20 mg	20 mg	75 mg
6	10 mg	10 mg	10 mg	10 mg	40 mg

In treatment settings where staff are less familiar with the assessment of alcohol withdrawal symptoms, an alternative approach is to prescribe a fixed-dose schedule of chlordiazepoxide 20–40 mg qds for 24–48 hours, with further prn doses of chlordiazepoxide 20–40 mg given for breakthrough withdrawal symptoms. After 48 hours, dose reductions by 20 per cent of the maximum prescribed dose can be prescribed as already detailed.

Supplementary prescribing in alcohol detoxification

Patients undergoing alcohol withdrawal may experience a number of uncomfortable symptoms. The primary treatment should be targeted at the alcohol withdrawal syndrome by the use of benzodiazepines. However, if other symptoms persist despite adequate treatment, supplementary symptomatic treatments can be used.

- *Pain/headaches:* paracetamol 1g prn, up to qds, can be used first line. Use caution with NSAIDs as many patients have gastritis or varices.
- *Nausea/vomiting:* prochlorperazine IM/po.
- *Hallucinations:* consider DTs and use additional chlordiazepoxide unless the patient is already sedated, in which case haloperidol 2–5 mg can be given prn up to 18 mg/24 hours.
- *Night sedation:* the evening dose of chlordiazepoxide prescribed for detoxification should provide a measure of night sedation. Benzodiazepines and benzodiazepine receptor agonists such as zopiclone and zolpidem should be avoided because of dependence potential. Patients complaining of chronic insomnia should be encouraged to learn non-pharmacological strategies. If supplementary prescribing for insomnia is essential, promethazine 25–50 mg nocte may be used.

Delirium tremens

Clinical features

Alcohol withdrawal phenomena: rapid onset of hallucinations, fear, disorientation, confusion, severe clouding of consciousness, tremor, tachycardia, fever, overactivity, and clamminess (all features not always present). The condition usually lasts for 3–5 days with gradual resolution, though it can be prolonged or life-threatening. Predisposing factors include hypoglycaemia, hypokalaemia, hypocalcaemia, and intercurrent infection.

Differential diagnosis

Delirium due to another cause, Wernicke's encephalopathy.

Management

The full-blown syndrome should be managed on the medical unit (mortality >5 per cent). Give adequate sedation (high doses of lorazepam or chlordiazepoxide, titrated until the patient is symptom-free and lightly sedated) and fluid replacement. Parenteral benzodiazepines (IM lorazepam) can be used if the patient is not able to take oral treatment. Because of the difficulty in reliably differentiating between DTs and Wernicke's encephalopathy, treatment for both conditions should be given (see the following). Beware withdrawal seizures. Once the patient has stabilized, benzodiazepines can be withdrawn over 5–10 days.

Wernicke's encephalopathy

Clinical features

The classic picture is of acute onset of nystagmus, gaze palsies, gait ataxia, and confusional state due to thiamine deficiency. It is most commonly seen in alcohol dependence, but may also occur in malnutrition and prolonged vomiting (including hyperemesis gravidarum, eating disorders, and self-neglect due to depression). Not all patients present with the classic picture; given the severe consequences of a missed diagnosis, one should have a low threshold for initiating treatment.

Differential diagnosis

Infective or metabolic encephalopathy, hydrocephalus, tumour, posterior circulation infarction, or haemorrhage.

Management
Treatment should be given as soon as the diagnosis is entertained, prefer-ably intravenously. This should be two pairs IM/IV ampoules high-potency B-complex vitamins three times daily for 3–5 days. If symptoms respond, continue one pair ampoules daily for 5 days or longer if improvement continues.

Alcohol-related seizures

Clinical features
Collapse, loss of consciousness, and seizure, usually occurring in the pres-ence of alcohol withdrawal—though up to 50 per cent of people who have an alcohol-related seizure will not report any recent change in their drinking patterns.

Differential diagnosis
Epilepsy, seizure due to other cause.

Management
A single seizure during detoxification can be managed by reviewing and optimizing chlordiazepoxide treatment and observing for 12–24 hours. Recurrent seizures require urgent admission to a medical unit and treat-ment with high-dose benzodiazepines (diazepam/chlordiazepoxide); diaze-pam 10 mg can be given PR while waiting for transfer. Phenytoin is not effective for alcohol withdrawal seizures and its use should be reserved for intractable seizures not responding to benzodiazepines or where there is uncertainty about the cause of the seizures.

Alcohol relapse prevention

After successful withdrawal, acamposate or oral naltrexone can be consid-ered, in combination with psychosocial intervention, to aid maintenance of abstinence. For harmful drinkers or those with mild dependence who have specifically requested pharmacological help, or for those where psychoso-cial interventions alone have not helped adequately, these medications can also be considered. See the British National Formulary (BNF) for prescrib-ing details.

Opioids

Opioids are drugs that principally interact with the mu opioid receptor, which is distributed in the brain, spinal cord, and gastrointestinal system. They are used clinically to control extreme distress (e.g. myocardial infarc-tion) and extreme pain. They produce euphoria, a sensation often described as being wrapped in 'emotional cotton wool'. A wide range of opioids may be misused; symptoms of intoxication and withdrawal vary in timing accord-ing to the plasma half-life (heroin < methadone < buprenorphine) and route of administration (oral > smoked (chased) > injected).

The opioid withdrawal syndrome
The effects of withdrawal from opioids are due to rebound high levels of central noradrenergic activity in the locus coeruleus and peripheral sym-pathetic autonomic activity. Onset depends upon the opioid used and the route administered, with onset between 12 and 72 hours, peak between

3 and 7 days, and milder effects such as sleep disturbance persisting for months. Symptoms include dysphoria, tachycardia, elevated blood pressure, pupillary dilation, rhinorrhoea, lacrymation, piloerection (goose pimples), nausea/vomiting, abdominal cramps, diarrhoea, skeletal muscle cramps, bone pain, anxiety. Masked underlying symptoms such as pain or emotional distress can be revealed. Craving for opioids and opioid-seeking behaviour are often the most marked withdrawal symptoms. Severity of symptoms is influenced by factors such as emotional state and the physical and social environment. Although markedly unpleasant, the withdrawal syndrome is not directly physically dangerous.

Opioid substitution therapy

The principle of opioid substitution therapy (OST) is to prescribe regular doses of an equivalent drug which acts at opioid receptors to replace the effects of heroin or other illicit drugs, prevent withdrawal symptoms, and, therefore, prevent the need for drug-seeking behaviour and associated harms. Harm reduction is as important an aim of treatment as abstinence. In time, once stabilized and engaged in appropriate psychosocial treatment, reduction in dose of the substituted opioid can be considered.

Substitute prescribing can take several forms:
• Short-term medically assisted withdrawal
• Longer-term (months) outpatient treatment, followed by detoxification once abstinent from illicit drugs
• Maintenance treatment in which the aim does not include detoxification except in the much longer term (years).

OST should usually be initiated in specialist addiction settings. Outpatient treatment should be initiated in community addiction services and should be closely supervised with regular key working and observed consumption of doses for several months until stabilized.

Patients attending emergency departments, GPs, or other community clinics claiming to have lost prescriptions or to be in opioid withdrawal should be directed to addiction services and not be given one-off prescriptions due to the high risk of diversion or double-dosing. Opioid withdrawal, though unpleasant, is not fatal; opioid overdose can be fatal.

However, if patients are admitted to hospital for medical or psychiatric treatment, opioids can be prescribed under supervision. Reasons include:
• continuation of already established therapy
• enabling the patient to remain in hospital for treatment rather than leaving to alleviate unpleasant withdrawal symptoms
• opportunistic initiation of OST with the aim of engagement in community treatment following discharge.

Advice can be sought from a local addiction specialist if necessary.
To continue already established therapy, confirm dose independently from community prescriber. Confirm last consumption supervised (e.g. from pharmacist). Patients who are also using heroin or street methadone of undetermined strength may report an overestimated dose for fear of being under-treated—administering an excessive dose based on patient report only may result in lethal overdose.

- If regular dose cannot be confirmed, initiate OST from starting dose.
- If last consumption unsupervised, initiate OST from starting dose.
- If more than 3 days have been missed, initiate OST from lower dose as tolerance may be lost.

Initiating opioid substitution therapy

Doctors unfamiliar with OST should prescribe under the guidance of an experienced clinician. If in doubt, do not prescribe, as opioid intoxication can kill, whereas opioid withdrawals do not.

First, establish that the patient is using and dependent on opioids. Methods include history taking, urine drug screening (note standard kits test for opioid and are not specific for heroin), inspection of injection sites, and examination for withdrawal symptoms.

Methadone, an opioid receptor agonist, and buprenorphine, an opioid receptor partial agonist, are licensed for OST. Buprenorphine is thought to reduce the risk of continuing 'on top' illicit drug use by partially blocking the effect of other opioids. In practice, there is little evidence of difference between the two. Methadone is considered first-line choice for OST, though patient preference should also be taken into account.

Note that methadone has a long half-life, which means that peak plasma concentration is not achieved for several days. Thus, overdose can be caused by both excessive starting doses and overly rapid titration.

Methadone can be initiated at 10–30 mg depending on tolerance (note that 20 mg is lethal in an opioid-naïve patient); if withdrawal symptoms persist, a further dose can be given by an experienced clinician within 6 hours but a total daily dose of 30–40 mg is generally enough to stop withdrawals. For the first 7 days after initiation, doses can be increased according to withdrawal symptoms by no more than 5–10 mg/day, to a maximum of 30 mg above the initial dose. Further increases should be by 5–10 mg and not exceed 30 mg/week. It is important to go slowly. Stabilization is usually achieved in 6 weeks but may take longer. Maintenance doses higher than 60 mg can be prescribed to suppress the benefits for patients of using heroin on top but this should be done by experienced clinicians only.

When initiating buprenorphine, the patient must already be in established opioid withdrawal to minimize the risk of precipitated withdrawal. Starting dose range is 2–8 mg depending on risk factors such as medical comorbidity, polysubstance misuse, low or uncertain dependence. 4 mg is a typical first dose. Further increases of 2–4 mg/day can be given until withdrawal symptoms are fully controlled. Maintenance doses are usually in the range 12–24 mg.

Be vigilant about prescribing either methadone or buprenorphine when other sedatives are in use (e.g. alcohol, benzodiazepines).

Aftercare

If OST is initiated in the inpatient setting, advance arrangements should be made for a community addiction service to take over prescribing. To minimize the risk of diversion or overdose, patients should not be given take-away supplies, but should be administered their dose on the morning of discharge and advised to attend the community service the same day for assessment. For newly initiated community prescriptions, patients are usually expected to collect daily supplies for supervised consumption until they have achieved 3 months' stability.

Opioid overdose

Excess opioids progressively produce difficulty in concentrating, confusion, intense sleepiness ('gouching' out), impaired rousability, respiratory depression, cyanosis, and coma. Opioid overdose is a major cause of death. Risk factors include fluctuations in purity of supply and changes in an individual's tolerance following a period of abstinence (e.g. on discharge from hospital, release from prison) or relapse. The triad of unrousability, cyanosis, and constricted pupils is virtually diagnostic of opioid overdose. Treatment is with the opioid antagonist naloxone 0.4 mg IV/IM and may need to be repeated if first dose does not work. Give high-flow oxygen, call an ambulance, and send to an acute medical hospital, even if apparently fully recovered. Naloxone has a short half-life (20 minutes) and can wear off before the opioid does, requiring infusion or repeat dosing in a hospital setting. As part of harm reduction, patients should be educated about the risks of overdose and trained in first aid to manage this situation in their friends. Take-away naloxone programmes can reduce death rates due to overdose.

Benzodiazepines and GABA-ergic drugs

Benzodiazepines, zopiclone, zolpidem, and related drugs act principally at GABA$_A$ receptors to potentiate the inhibitory effects of GABA, resulting in reduced anxiety and feelings of calm, comfort, and somnolence. In addition to illicit use, iatrogenic dependence is common following long-term prescription. As a treatment for anxiety, benzodiazepines are licensed for short-term use only. Tolerance may develop with regular use, resulting in the emergence of withdrawal symptoms despite regular dosing; if these symptoms are misinterpreted as emergence of anxiety, then the prescriber may escalate the dose rather than considering alternative treatments.

Benzodiazepine withdrawal

Benzodiazepines have a wide range of half-lives which affect the pattern and severity of onset and withdrawal. Short-acting drugs such as lorazepam or temazepam are associated with more withdrawal problems than longer-acting drugs like diazepam or clonazepam. The emergence of withdrawal symptoms may have an acute or insidious onset in this situation and, with diazepam, may occur several days after the last dose. Symptoms are due to reduced activity of the GABA inhibitory complex and excess glutamatergic drive. The predominant picture is that of anxiety. Other features include severe dysphoria/restlessness, tachycardia, tachypnoea, nausea, tightness in chest or abdomen, tight/aching muscles, fine tremor, and perceptual distortion. The insidious and subtle nature of symptoms can make them difficult to distinguish from other conditions such as anxiety disorders and opioid withdrawal. However, they are often marked by desperate attempts to obtain further supplies. Despite concern about risk of seizures, the rate is substantially lower than for alcohol withdrawal.

Prescribing for benzodiazepine dependence

Unlike opioid substitution therapy, there is little evidence of benefit from routine prescribing of benzodiazepines as maintenance treatment for dependence. Detoxification and maintenance therapy should be reserved for specialist addiction services. In an inpatient mental health setting, the clinical picture is often complicated by the presence of comorbid anxiety or personality disorders. If severe withdrawal symptoms occur, then it may be necessary to prescribe diazepam to relieve distress, then taper over 7–20 days. Maintenance prescribing after discharge should only be considered in agreement with a community addiction service. Principles of prescribing include:

- Always confirm reported dose with previous prescriber, to avoid risk of overdose due to dose exaggeration.
- Prescribe, as far as possible, according to objective withdrawal symptoms.
- Aim to consolidate multiple benzodiazepines into prescribing a single drug, usually diazepam.
- Focus on longer-term treatment of underlying anxiety or personality disorders, e.g. using antidepressants or psychological therapies rather than benzodiazepines.
- Use anxiolytics with less dependence potential, e.g. the sedating antihistamines promethazine or hydroxyzine.
- If discharge on maintentance diazepam is considered, the maximum dose that should be used is 30 mg daily.
- Ensure that the risks of double-scripting are minimized by regular communication between primary care, mental health, and addiction services. Daily dispensed doses are recommended unless stability confirmed.

Benzodiazepine overdose

Overdose symptoms include confusion, loss of consciousness, slowing of reflexes, incoordination, 'paradoxical' disinhibition, respiratory depression, and unconsciousness. The sedative effects are increased by opioids and alcohol. Overdose is a medical emergency and the patient should be given high-flow oxygen, airway support, and transferred to hospital. The specific antagonist, flumazenil, may be used to reverse overdose (1–3 mg IV), though with caution in overdoses of unknown quantity or substance as it may precipitate seizures.

Cocaine, amphetamines, and other stimulant drugs

Stimulants include cocaine and amphetamines (including methamphetamine). They are usually snorted or swallowed, though 'crack' cocaine is smoked and both cocaine and amphetamines can be injected. All stimulate release of monoamines, principally dopamine, to produce euphoria.

Stimulant-induced confusion and anxiety states

Stimulants can be used repeatedly until exhaustion, physical or financial, supervenes. However, their use can cause acute effects which can be severe enough to present to the general psychiatrist. These states are commonly of euphoria or anxiety, but may proceed to more severe symptoms such as paranoid ideation leading to violent and aggressive behaviour and auditory or visual hallucinations. Insight is usually retained or only transiently impaired. Management involves calming and reassuring the patient until the effects wear off. Occasionally, hospital admission and treatment with oral diazepam (10–20 mg) may be needed and, in severe cases, antipsychotic medication is required.

Stimulant withdrawal

When stopped abruptly, stimulants produce a brief physical withdrawal syndrome or 'crash', marked by exhaustion, depressed mood, and motivation. Trials of various medications have found these to be of little value, and most patients just need advice regarding the likely symptoms, reassurance that they will pass, and a safe place to get through this period. Some patients may become acutely suicidal and will require hospital admission and close observation. A short course of chlordiazepoxide may help relieve severe withdrawal symptoms in the inpatient setting, e.g. 40 mg qds (day 1), 30 mg qds (day 2), 20 mg qds (day 3), 10 mg qds (day 4), though should be avoided in outpatient settings.

Hallucinogens and empathogens

Drugs such as LSD, psilocybin (magic mushrooms) and 3,4-methylenedioxymethamphetamine (MDMA or ecstasy) do not produce a physical withdrawal syndrome and can be stopped abruptly. One crucial exception is ketamine (Special K), a dissociative anaesthetic causing psychedelic experiences that may produce dependence. Some people experience severe psychological distress during or after use of hallucinogens and may need a safe place to be while the experience passes, and, occasionally, symptomatic treatment such as a brief course of benzodiazepines to reduce anxiety.

Gamma-butyrolactone (GBL) and gamma-hydroxybutyrone (GHB)

These solvents are taken orally in drops or mixed with water and potentiate GABA neurotransmission to cause central nervous system depression, producing euphoria and disinhibition in low doses. The window of effect is narrow and easily misjudged: overdose results in collapse and respiratory depression, and is treated by respiratory support until the drug is eliminated. The short half-life and rapid development of tolerance result in a high potential for dependence; dependent users often describe having to stay awake to dose every 2–4 hours around the clock. The withdrawal syndrome begins with tachycardia, fine tremor, sweating, and severe dysphoria/anxiety, and progresses to a state of severe agitated delirium. In some cases, muscle rigidity and rhabdomyolysis develops, and fatalities have been reported.

Elective detoxification should be undertaken in specialist addiction treatment services. GBL/GHB withdrawal should be suspected and enquired about if someone presents to the emergency department in a state of severe agitation which does not respond to initial doses of sedatives. Patients in established withdrawal should be admitted to a medical ward for management with high doses of diazepam and baclofen. In severe cases, sedation in the intensive care unit may be required.

Further reading

Taylor, D., Paton, C., and Kapur, S. (2012). *The Maudsley Prescribing Guidelines in Psychiatry*. 11th Edition. Wiley-Blackwell.

Bell, J. and Collins, R. (2011). Gamma-butyrolactone (GBL) dependence and withdrawal. *Addiction*, 106(2), 442–7.

Psychotherapy

All patients referred to a psychiatrist should receive psychological consideration, even if the primary treatment is medication. Selected patients can be referred onwards for specialist assessment and treatment which, in the NHS, usually means psychodynamic, cognitive–behavioural, short-term psychodynamic, or systemic (family/couple) therapy. Where referral for specialist psychotherapy is not appropriate, psychotherapeutic principles can still inform management and psychotherapists can still contribute to case discussion. The main criteria for patient referral are someone who is motivated to understand his/her difficulties in psychological terms and who can contain his/her anxiety without behaving in unmanageably destructive ways.

Psychodynamic psychotherapy

In considering who might benefit from this kind of therapy, diagnosis is less important than personal characteristics. Thus, someone who wishes to address problems in the context of a relationship, who is not aiming for immediate symptom relief, and who can tolerate the relatively unstructured setting necessary for the optimal exploration of personal difficulties might benefit from this approach. There are no absolute contraindications but, in practice, active drug or alcohol misuse, active psychosis, or a significant tendency towards self-harm or violence would preclude treatment in standard NHS facilities. Most people treated have neurotic or personality problems (e.g. depression, anxiety, difficulties with partners, friends, or peers, problems with loss and interdependence), which they inevitably reproduce with the therapist, allowing them to be worked with in a 'live' way. Both individual and group treatments are usually available, with the choice depending on a balance of factors including patient preference.

Cognitive–behavioural therapy (CBT)

The premise behind this therapy is that thoughts, actions, emotions, and physiology influence one another in a cyclical fashion, and that intervening at any point of the cycle can productively disrupt it. Thus, depression is characterized by a negative thought pattern about self, the world, and the future, and can be treated by challenging these thoughts, as well as physiologically (by medication) or behaviourally (by a programme of activity). In cognitive therapy, the emphasis is on challenging dysfunctional thinking, although in practice most programmes include a behavioural component. The main criteria for suitability are that the model makes sense to the patient and that s/he is willing to experiment with alternative ways of thinking both in the sessions and between them, as 'homework'.

As with other forms of therapy, the patient has to be able to contain anxiety sufficiently to work within the model. However, the more structured nature of the sessions and their more conscious content render CBT inherently less anxiety-provoking than psychodynamic therapy. CBT has been shown to be effective in depression, anxiety, phobias, and obsessive–compulsive and eating disorders, among others. In addition, some aspects of psychosis are amenable to CBT and, less commonly, the techniques have been used in groups. People with personality disorders may respond to longer-term, more specialized CBT, although psychodynamic therapy is often the preferred option in these cases. CBT principles also form the basis of several self-help approaches including computer-based psychotherapies.

Family therapy

Unlike most other therapies, useful work can be done in these sessions even when the index patient is too ill to participate fully. This is because resultant shifts in the family system may operate to the patient's (as well as the family's) benefit. Moreover, the more ill the patient, the more the family is entitled to consideration in its own right, especially as family members may be involved in long-term care and support. A great deal can be gained by making a family dynamic assessment early on in treatment, and, in principle, any family that expresses a willingness to work together with a skilled professional in helping their ill member is suitable for referral for family therapy. Family therapy has been shown to be effective in reducing relapse in schizophrenia, as well as in adolescent anorexia nervosa, and as a couple treatment for depression where one partner is affected. In family therapy, no clear distinction is made between assessment and therapy; the first session aims to establish a treatment contract and this contract is reviewed regularly. In practice, a typical contract might involve four to six sessions over a 2–3 month period, depending on response.

Case discussion

Psychotherapists can offer discussion of complicated cases, even when these are unlikely to be suitable for psychotherapy. This can happen as a one-off or as part of a regular seminar attended by all members of the multidisciplinary team. In practice, these seminars tend to be offered by psychodynamically oriented therapists, who are trained to think about the dynamics evoked in the team as well as about the individual patient. The patients discussed tend to be the ones who generate most emotion and controversy among those trying to help them and often suffer from a personality disorder. Case discussions help the staff to keep track of counter-transference interference with sound judgement and good management.

Mental health law

The law puts various duties on health systems and professionals to support individuals, including people with mental disorder, to make decisions about their own health whilst respecting their choices. This is 'supported' decision making. However, the law also recognizes that people with mental disorder may, at times, require others to decide their health care. This is 'substitute' decision making. In England and Wales, there are two main substitute decision-making frameworks for people who are seeing a psychiatrist: the Mental Health Act 1983 (MHA) and the Mental Capacity Act 2005 (MCA). Each is based on different principles. The MHA is restricted to compulsory treatment for mental disorder whilst the MCA has a broader scope, applying to physical and mental health as well as to welfare, finances, property, and research participation.

This chapter summarizes the MHA and the MCA frameworks and outlines some other statutory schemes of relevance for the psychiatrist.

Mental Health Act 1983

The Act applies to patients of any age. The Code of Practice (revised 2008) begins with a statement of guiding principles that although not included in the Act itself, should inform decisions. The 'purpose principle' states a utilitarian ideal that decisions under the Act must be taken with a view to minimizing the undesirable effects of mental disorder, by maximizing the safety and well-being (mental and physical) of patients, promoting their recovery, and protecting other people from harm. Other principles are:

- the least restriction principle
- the respect principle
- the patient participation principle
- the effectiveness, efficiency, and equity principle.

Some guidance on applying these principles is given in the Code of Practice.

Criteria for compulsory treatment in those with mental disorder

Mental disorder is defined by the Act as 'any disorder or disability of the mind'. This broad definition is intended to include personality disorder. The only psychiatric disorder that is not considered a mental disorder by the MHA is dependence on alcohol or drugs. Patients with learning disability are excluded from longer-term detention or guardianship unless they have abnormally aggressive or seriously irresponsible conduct. The law looks to objective medical evidence in determining mental disorder.

As well as satisfying the criterion for mental disorder, a person must meet the criteria in Box 10.1.

Mental Health Act assessments

If the person is subject to the effects of sedative medication or the short-term effects of drugs or alcohol, Mental Health Act assessment should wait until the effects have abated, unless this is not possible because of the patient's disturbed behaviour.

Box 10.1 Criteria for compulsory treatment in those with mental disorder

1. The mental disorder is of a nature* or degree which warrants detention, *and*
2. The compulsory treatment is in the interests of his/her own health, **or** safety, **or** for the protection of other persons.

* Nature is usually interpreted as referring to the historical pattern of the disorder and degree to the present mental state. Although suicide and violence may dominate interpretations of the interests (or risk) criteria, it is important to note that health is also covered (including mental health).

Source: The MHA (1983) and Code of Practice

Except for emergencies, two independent doctors and an **approved mental health professional** (AMHP) make assessments and consensus is required for detention to be authorized. If consensus cannot be reached, effort should be made to gain more information or devise an alternative plan rather than abandon the patient.

Applications typically follow referral to the AMHP. The AMHP is responsible for coordinating the process of assessment, implementing the decision for application, speaking to the nearest relative, communicating the decision to the patient and relevant parties, and conveying the patient to hospital.

The **doctor** is responsible for the following:

1. Carrying out a direct personal examination of the patient's mental state, and obtaining and considering all available relevant medical information.
2. Ensuring that a hospital bed is available if needed.

The Code of Practice stipulates that, in every case, regard should be had to:

- The patient's current wishes and views of their own needs.
- Past wishes or feelings expressed by the patient.
- The patient's age and physical health.
- The patient's cultural background.
- The patient's social and family circumstances.
- The impact that any future deterioration or lack of improvement in the patient's condition would have on their children, other relatives, or carers, especially those living with the patient, including an assessment of these people's ability and willingness to cope.
- The effect on the patient, and those close to the patient, of a decision to admit or not to admit under the Act.

Before it is decided that admission to hospital is necessary, consideration must be given to whether there are alternative means of providing the care and treatment that the patient requires. This includes consideration of whether there might be other effective forms of care or treatment the patient would be willing to accept.

Wherever possible, the doctors and AMHPs should consult colleagues (e.g. community psychiatric nurses (CPNs), GPs), carers, and family members, but they retain final responsibility.

Common orders for civil patients

Admission for assessment (Section 2)

This is for up to 28 days and may include treatment following assessment.
The Code of Practice states that Section 2 should be preferred where:

(a) The full extent of the nature and degree of a patient's condition is unclear.
(b) There is a need to carry out an initial inpatient assessment in order to formulate a treatment plan or to reach a judgement about whether the patient will accept treatment on a voluntary basis following admission: or
(c) There is a need to carry out a new inpatient assessment in order to re-formulate a treatment plan or to reach a judgement about whether the patient will accept treatment on a voluntary basis.

Admission for treatment (Section 3)

This is for up to 6 months and renewable.
The Code of Practice states that Section 3 should be preferred where:

(a) The patient is already detained under Section 2 (detention under Section 2 cannot be renewed by another Section 2 application): or
(b) The nature and current degree of the patient's mental disorder, the essential elements of the treatment plan to be followed, and the likelihood of the patient accepting treatment on a voluntary basis are already established.

Mentally disordered persons found in public places (Section 136)

This is a police power to remove a person found in public who appears to be suffering from a mental disorder and in immediate need of care and control to a place of safety. 'Place of safety' is defined quite broadly. The power authorizes detention for up to 72 hours for the purpose of enabling assessment by a doctor and an AMHP.

Admission for treatment in cases of emergency (Section 4)

This is a power, to be used only in cases of urgent necessity, to admit a person compulsorily for assessment for up to 72 hours. It requires application by an AMHP or nearest relative and one medical recommendation (who need not be S12 approved). The same criteria for Section 2 apply and there must be evidence for why obtaining a second medical recommendation would cause undesirable delay.

Holding powers for informally admitted patients (Section 5)

A registered doctor in charge of a patient's inpatient treatment or another doctor they nominate (e.g. an on-call doctor) can hold a person for up to 72 hours to enable a Section 2 or Section 3 assessment. This is a Section 5(2) power and may apply in a psychiatric or a general hospital but not an A&E department. A first-level registered mental health nurse has a similar holding power of 6 hours, which might be a necessary first step before a Section 5(2) assessment.

Supervised community treatment/community treatment order (CTO)

These are a new legal intervention in England and Wales and may be initiated only when a patient is being treated under Section 3 (or Section

37, see following details). The criteria for eligibility are similar to Section 3. Community treatment, with a liability to be recalled to hospital if the patient fails to comply with a condition of the CTO, replaces inpatient treatment.

The treatment conditions cannot be enforced in the community but the patient may be recalled to hospital. Once a patient arrives at hospital under recall, they may be detained for a maximum of 72 hours whilst the responsible clinician (RC) determines what should happen next. If the RC decides to revoke the CTO and treat in hospital beyond 72 hours, this requires the agreement of an AMHP. Revoking a CTO does not cancel a CTO but merely puts it in the background; it brings back the powers of the initial Section 3 (or 37) for 6 months and triggers a Mental Health Tribunal (MHT) referral. If the CTO is not revoked, the patient may return to the community where the CTO powers remain in place. CTOs may be renewed in the community. Initial extension lasts 6 months and, thereafter, 12 months. Application to the MHT can be made by a patient whilst in the community. Three randomized controlled trials (RCTs), with 6–12 month follow-up, have not shown effectiveness.

Common orders for patients involved in criminal proceedings (Part III of the MHA)

Hospital order (Section 37)

The **duration** is initially for 6 months and is renewable for a further 6 months, and then yearly. The **procedure** is as follows. The order can be made by a Crown or Magistrates' Court in the case of a convicted offender in place of a prison sentence (offences include manslaughter but not murder). The Magistrates' Court need not record a conviction if satisfied that the offender was suffering from mental disorder at the time of the offence. In all other respects, it operates like a Section 3.

Restriction order (Section 41)

The **duration** may be specified by court or without limit. The **procedure** is as follows. The order can be made by a Crown Court only after imposition of a hospital order (Section 37) if:
- this is necessary to protect the public from 'serious harm' *and*
- at least one of the doctors who made recommendations for the hospital order gave evidence orally.

RCs have no power to rescind this section. Tribunals may absolutely discharge patients from the restriction order but decisions are open to challenge by the Home Secretary.

A note on Mental Health Tribunals (MHTs)

A patient detained is entitled to apply to a MHT to contest the lawfulness of detention. Hospital managers also have various duties to refer cases. The MHT is, in effect, a court whose task is to determine whether, at the time of the hearing, the criteria justifying detention continue to be met. The court, chaired by a legal member, expects written and oral evidence from the treating team to address the criteria for detention.

A note on ECT

The MHA has a new rule that incapacity to decide ECT is a necessary (though not sufficient) criterion for ECT to be given compulsorily. Included in this are the MCA rules on anticipatory decision making (see 'Anticipatory decision making', p. 168). If, however, the compulsory ECT is needed to save the patient's life or is immediately necessary to prevent serious deterioration to his or her condition (Section 62), then incapacity is not a necessary criterion. For detained patients without capacity, or under 18, ECT requires the approval of a second-opinion doctor (SOAD).

A note on informal patients

The MHA states that nothing in the Act prohibits informal treatment in hospital—that is, treatment without detention. Some of these patients who are not detained will have capacity to decide treatment and some will not. It is thus important to assess capacity in the informal group, if there are concerns. This is to ensure that the best interests of a person admitted informally, but without capacity to decide treatment (e.g. some people with dementia or severe depression), are being identified and acted on (see 'Best interests', p. 167), that there are safeguards for patients deprived of their liberty (see 'Deprivation of Liberty Safeguards and Deprivation of Liberty', p. 169), or that coercion is not occurring in a person with capacity to decide treatment. See Table 10.1 for ways detained patients become informal patients.

Mental Capacity Act 2005

The MCA is a relatively new Act that codifies a lot of pre-existing common law. It may apply when the MHA is not being used and it interplays, in various ways, with the MHA. The Act applies to persons age 16 and over. It has five principles on the face of the statute emphasizing an ideal of personal autonomy.

1. A person must be assumed to have capacity unless it is established that they lack capacity.
2. A person is not to be treated as unable to make a decision unless all practicable steps to help him/her to do so have been taken, without success.
3. A person is not to be treated as unable to make a decision merely because s/he makes an unwise decision
4. An act done or a decision made, under this Act, for or on behalf of a person who lacks capacity, must be done or made in his/her best interests.
5. Before the act is done or the decision is made, regard must be had to whether the purpose for which it is needed can be as effectively achieved in a way that is less restrictive of the person's rights and freedoms of action.

There are three basic concepts in the MCA: decision-making capacity, best interests, and anticipatory decision making.

Table 10.1 Discharge possibilities under the Mental Health Act 1983

Section	Discharge
2—Admission for assessment	By any of the following: (a) Decision of the RC (b) Lapse of 28 days without application for S3 (c) Decision of hospital managers (d) Request of the nearest relative who must give 72 hours' notice; RC can prevent nearest relative discharging patient by making a report to hospital managers. (e) Decision of MHT: patient can apply to a tribunal within the first 14 days of detention.
3—Admission for treatment	By any of the following: (a) Decision of the RC (b) Disagreement between RC and a second professional about renewal of Section 3 in the 2 months prior to Section 3 expiry (unless exceptional circumstances) or disagreement between RC and hospital managers about extension of Section 3. (c) Decision of hospital managers (d) Request of nearest relative (as for Section 2 above) (e) Decision of MHT: patient can apply to a tribunal within 6 months of admission and during each subsequent renewal period.
17—Community Treatment Orders	By any of the following: (a) Decision of the RC (b) Disagreement between the RC and a second professional about renewal of CTO in the 2 months prior to CTO expiry (unless exceptional circumstances) or disagreement between RC and AMHP about extension of CTO. (c) Nearest relatives—if person detained in hospital (see Section 3 above) (d) Decision of hospital managers (e) Decision of MHT

RC, Responsible Clinician; AMHP, Approved Mental Health Professional; 'Second Professional', a professional concerned with the medical treatment of the person who belongs to a profession other than that of the RC; MHT, Mental Health Tribunal

Decision-making capacity (DMC)

The MCA presumes ability to decide, but when there are appropriate concerns, requires assessment of DMC. The assessment determines whether a health-care professional needs to act in an individual's best interests (see 'Best interests', p. 167) or in a way that respects informed, freely given choice as the person's own.

The MCA frames DMC as a test of the impact of a mental disorder on a specific decision-making process that faces a person (e.g. a health decision, a residential decision). It tests ability to decide in terms of both an ability to understand relevant information and an ability to make decisions on the basis of that understanding (see Box 10.2).

Assessment of DMC is not a test of a person's status (such as soundness of mind or diagnosis) or of the eccentricity of someone's decision (such as a refusal of a conventional treatment). DMC can fluctuate over time and is dependent on the decision at hand. For example, a person with Alzheimer's disease may have problems understanding, retaining, and weighing information about treatment, whereas one with severe depression or schizophrenia may have problems understanding and using that information in the process of deciding. The test thus covers the decision-making problems people with mental disorders of any kind may have, without assuming that these problems affect all their decisions. Box 10.3 gives an approach to DMC assessment. Research has shown incapacity for health-care decision making to be common in acute wards of general hospitals, with rates fairly similar to those of mental health hospitals, but with different underlying causes. In medical inpatient settings, there is a tendency for incapacity to go unrecognized and to be considered only when there is treatment refusal.

Box 10.2 The two-stage test of decision-making capacity

Stage 1

Does the person have an impairment of, or a disturbance in the functioning of, the mind or brain? (It does not matter whether it is temporary or permanent.)

Stage 2

If so, does that impairment or disturbance mean that the person is unable to make the decision in question at the time it needs to be made?
    Inability means inability to:
- understand the information relevant to the decision
- retain that information
- use or weigh that information as part of the process of making the decision
- communicate any decision (whether by talking, using sign language, or any other means).

Source: The MCA Code of Practice (2005)

Box 10.3 An approach to decision-making capacity assessment

Before the interview

- What is it that the person needs to decide about (e.g. treatment, residence, financial affairs, legal proceedings)?
- Do I understand what needs deciding about well enough to communicate the right kind of information?
- What is the level of urgency and what are the implications of refusal?
- What is the psychopathology and how should the interview be guided by this?
- Are there some concrete, specific issues that must be raised at the interview (e.g. a previous change of mind in relation to the decision, a risky behaviour)?
- What information has s/he been given?
- Are there barriers to understanding (language, communication)?
- Who are the patient's social supports?

During the interview

- Aim to communicate what needs to be understood and aim to understand your patient's decision making and its relation to the psychopathology.
- Keep the decision in mind.
- Be willing to engage the person about who usually helps them make decisions.
- In treatment refusals, where the patient is protesting because they feel angry, undermined, or anxious, give plenty of chances for cooling down and face-saving ways to reverse refusal.

After the interview

- Discuss with other members of the clinical team, relatives, GP (plus anyone else relevant).
- Keep good records.
- In difficult cases, try to let time resolve disputes if possible, be willing to have another go or seek a second opinion, or seek further legal advice (e.g. trust legal department, emergency access to court).

Best interests

The MCA does not define 'best interests' but, rather, provides a set of checks on the process of deciding what they are (see Box 10.4). In relation to health care, best interests aims to implement three basic ideas:
1. Treatment for the person should be the least restrictive of liberty.
2. Treatment should be for the benefit of the patient.
3. Treatment should aim to be what the person would have wanted if they had had capacity to decide.

If the treatment the person would have wanted can be discovered indirectly (e.g. through friends/family or an independent mental capacity advocate),

Box 10.4 Checklist for best interests

- Working out what is in a person's best interests cannot be based simply on age, appearance, condition, or behaviour.
- *All relevant circumstances should be considered when working out best interests.*
- *Every effort should be made to encourage and enable a person who lacks capacity to take part in making the decision.*
- *If there is a chance that a person will regain the capacity to make a particular decision, then it may be possible to put it off until later if it is not urgent.*
- When the determination relates to life-sustaining treatment, the best interests decision maker (e.g. the doctor) must not, in considering whether the treatment is in the best interests of the person concerned, be motivated by a desire to bring about his/her death.
- *A person's past and present wishes and feelings, beliefs, and values should be taken into account.*
- *The views of other people who are close to the person who lacks capacity should be considered, as well as those of an attorney or deputy.*

N.B. Italics indicate checks considered by the editors to be most relevant to doctors.
Source: The MCA (2005) and Code of Practice

this should have influence in identifying best interests, as should the present feelings and beliefs of the person. Best interests assessment emphasizes process and aims to place a check on any health-care decision makers 'I know best' instinct or on any tendency to assume that family members can consent for an incapable adult.

Decisions taken according to best interests for persons without DMC are protected from liability (i.e. legal action taken against the doctor). Restraint is authorized in best interests if the restrainer believes it is necessary and the restraint is in proportion to the harm otherwise faced by the person. Confinement will raise the question of deprivation of liberty (see 'Deprivation of Liberty Safeguards and Deprivation of Liberty', p. 169).

In true emergency situations, where there may be uncertainty about DMC or time does not allow the best interest checklist to be worked through, the MCA defaults to saving life.

Anticipatory decision making

One of the ways the MCA aims to enable autonomous decision making is to encourage people's planning of their health care for times when capacity to decide is lost. When a person has capacity to decide, they do not have a legal right to determine what treatment a doctor recommends but they do have a right to refuse a treatment recommended. The MCA recognizes an extension of these rights to **future** situations of incapacity. A person can state advance preferences **for** certain kinds of treatment and make advance **refusals** of treatment. Only advances refusals are legally binding, although a best interests decision maker can jettison them if there is evidence that they are not valid (e.g. made without DMC, insufficiently informed, coerced) or applicable (e.g. not relating to the decision the best interest assessor is facing). Advanced refusals of life-sustaining treatment need to be signed and witnessed.

Another form of anticipatory decision making is appointment of a lasting power of attorney (LPA) for health care. This is a new legal intervention in England and Wales. A person can nominate a relation or friend (one or more) to become their attorney for health (a somewhat similar legal responsibility to being a 'responsible parent' in the Children Act (see 'Children Act 1989', p. 170)). This makes the attorney the legal best interests decision maker for health and creates a doctor–patient relationship that is legally mediated by a third party. The impact of this new power has yet to be felt on the ground. In the USA, where health-care proxies exist in most jurisdictions, research has shown that proxies, when appointed by capable adults, predict patient treatment preferences with around 68 per cent accuracy.

Anticipatory decision making applies to adults only (18 and above). It has no legal force in the MHA, although the patient participation principle emphasizes the role of the patient in the planning, developing, and reviewing of their own treatment.

Deprivation of Liberty Safeguards and Deprivation of Liberty

Deprivation of Liberty Safeguards (DoLS) were inserted into the MCA after it became an Act of Parliament and should be distinguished from 'Deprivation of Liberty' which refers to a basic right in the European Convention on Human Rights (Article 5). DoLS attempts to plug the 'Bournewood Gap'—the category of persons who lack capacity, are deprived of their liberty, but are not detained under the MHA. The current eligibility criteria for DoLS are obscure and unreliably judged by experts. Whilst this remains the case, giving practical guidance on DoLS is beset with difficulties. Recent judgements have directed its application towards cases involving dementia and learning disability in care homes.

The distinction between 'restriction of liberty' and 'deprivation of liberty' is a matter of degree, but any 'deprivation of liberty' needs a formal safeguarding procedure (e.g. DoLS or MHA). Box 10.5 gives the criteria for deprivation of liberty. If you think a deprivation of liberty might be occurring without safeguards (e.g. in a care home for people with dementia or learning disabilities), then consider with the care team:

1) whether the level of restriction of liberty is actually in best interests and whether it can be reduced
2) whether a referral to the local authority for a DoLS assessment is required
3) whether a MHA assessment is needed.

Box 10.5 Deprivation of liberty criteria
1) Confinement imputable to the state (e.g. carried out in hospitals, care homes).
2) Confinement to a certain limited place for a not negligible length of time (not free to leave the place they are living and under continuous supervision and control).
3) The person has not validly consented to the confinement (they have objected, have consented without being sufficiently informed, have lacked DMC, or have been coerced).

Sources: *Storck v Germany* [2005] 43 EHRR 96; Cheshire West and Chester Council v P (2014) UKSC 19

Safeguarding vulnerable adults

Case law has defined the 'vulnerable adult' as a person who is or may be in need of community care services by reason of mental or other disability, age, or illness, and who is or may be unable to take care of him or herself against **significant harm or exploitation**. It may include adults with or without mental capacity.

The responsibility for safeguarding vulnerable adults lies with local authority social services. Referral should be made urgently to adult safeguarding teams and/or to the police if abuse is thought to be occurring. For other referrals, 'significant harm' is best interpreted using common sense. The safeguarding teams have duties to investigate and authority to share information, on a need-to-know basis, between health, social service, police, and other agencies. The aim is to put in place plans to protect vulnerable adults and review the effectiveness of those plans.

Children Act 1989

This Act applies to any child (below age 18). The central principle is that the welfare of the child is paramount. This principle of welfare is similar to the best interests principle in the MCA but has a slightly different checklist. In child law, capacity is not presumed in the under 16s. A maturity-based concept of 'Gillick competence' exists for the under 16s and, if competent, a doctor can accept the consent of the child. However, an absolute right to refuse treatment does not exist in the under 18s. The key concept is 'parental responsibility'. A person with parental responsibility has the legal authority to decide treatment for the child (its proxy) and so must be identified and consulted. A biological mother automatically has parental responsibility, as does a biological father if married to the mother. Parental responsibility can be lost and acquired (e.g. for children in care). The person with parental responsibility can consent to, or refuse, treatment for the child, even if against the child's wishes, if consistent with the child's welfare. Use of the MHA becomes appropriate if compulsion is required for treatment of mental disorder.

Safeguarding children

Local authorities have the duty to safeguard and promote the welfare of children in need and, so far as is consistent with that duty, to promote the upbringing of children within their families. Thus, referral of children with needs to the local authority (children and families safeguarding teams) can often be done consensually as a way of releasing services for the child. This can be important in adult mental health services when a parent's mental illness, or environment, is impacting on the health and development of their child or children.

If there is reasonable cause to suspect that a child is suffering, or is likely to suffer, **significant harm** to his/her health or development, referral to the local authority must be made quickly and does not require consent. Local authorities can seek emergency protection orders from courts. Criminal proceedings can proceed in parallel if there are abuse offenses.

Children and family teams in local authorities often build up a picture of harm to a child (which they must investigate if judged significant) by receiving referrals from different agencies at different times (e.g. a GP treating the child, adult mental health services treating a parent, teachers at the child's school). Each agency may be unaware of the other's referrals, so logging concerns about harm may be important even if you are uncertain about the **significant harm** threshold and even if the child and families team do not immediately investigate your referral.

Police and Criminal Evidence Act 1984

Parts of this Act deal with the treatment and questioning of people with mental disorder in police custody. If a person in custody appears mentally disordered (defined according to MHA criteria), police must ask an 'appropriate adult' to come to the police station. Concern is that people with mental disorder will give evidence which is unreliable and/or self-incriminatory. This does not apply in emergencies (e.g. where risk to others can be reduced by questioning someone immediately).

The 'appropriate adult' can be a relative, a carer, or someone who has worked with the mentally disordered, but it cannot be the person's solicitor. The adult cannot be employed by the police. The Code of Practice states that a well-informed professional may be preferable to an ill-informed relative, but also that the person's choice of adult is to be respected.

The 'appropriate adult' should be present during searches and questioning, observe fairness of interviews, advise the person being questioned, and facilitate communication. The person being questioned is entitled to consult privately with the appropriate adult at any time.

The Care Programme Approach

The Care Programme Approach (CPA) was introduced in 1991 and is a quasi legal system aiming to guide good clinical practice and to prevent patients from 'slipping through the net'. The key principles are applicable to all service users.

Its four main elements are as follows:

1. **Assessment of health and social care needs.**
2. **A written care plan:** agreed as far as possible with the patient and with carers.
3. **Care coordinator:** has responsibility for the coordination of the care programme. S/he is responsible for keeping in close contact with the patient, and for advising the other members of the care team of changes in the circumstances of the patient which might require review or modification of the care plan. The care coordinator should be the professional with the closest relationship with the patient; this will often be a CPN or social worker, but could be a psychiatrist in training.
4. **Ongoing reviews:** review and evaluation of care planning should be regarded as an ongoing process. There is no required set period for review but, at each review meeting, the date of the next review must be set and recorded. Any member of the care team, or the patient or carer, must be able to ask for a review at any time. If the team decides that a review is not necessary, the reasons for this must be recorded.

Who should receive the CPA?

The characteristics of patients who should receive the CPA are those with severe mental disorder (including personality disorder) where there is a high degree of complexity. For example:

- multiple care needs, including unsettled accommodation, employment problems, etc., requiring inter-agency coordination
- contact with a number of agencies
- coexisting substance misuse or learning disabilities
- more likely to be at risk of harming themselves or others
- more likely to disengage with services
- currently/recently detained under MHA, on CTO, or referred to crisis/home treatment team
- significant reliance on carer/s or has own caring responsibilities.

Psychiatrists work in a complex legal space requiring adherence to increasing amounts of legislation. Trainees should discuss cases with multidisciplinary colleagues and with seniors as they are learning the law.

Further reading

Fennell, P. (2011). *Mental Health: The New Law (2nd Edition).* Jordans.
Hale, B. (2010). *Mental Health Law (5th Edition).* Sweet and Maxwell.

The AUDIT questionnaire

Circle the number that comes closest to the patient's answer.[1]

1. How often do you have a drink containing alcohol?

(0) Never   (1) Monthly or less
(2) 2–4 times a month   (3) 2–3 times a week
(4) 4 or more times a week

2.[a] How many drinks containing alcohol do you have on a typical day
when you are drinking? (Code number of standard drinks)

(0) 1 or 2   (1) 3 or 4   (2) 5 or 6
(3) 7 or 8   (4) 10 or more

3. How often do you have six or more drinks on one occasion?

(0) Never   (1) Less than monthly   (2) Monthly
(3) Weekly   (4) Daily or almost daily

4. How often during the past year have you found that you were not able
to stop drinking once you had started?

(0) Never   (1) Less than monthly   (2) Monthly
(3) Weekly   (4) Daily or almost daily

5. How often during the past year have you failed to do what was
normally expected from you because of drinking?

(0) Never   (1) Less than monthly   (2) Monthly
(3) Weekly   (4) Daily or almost daily

6. How often during the past year have you needed a first drink in the
morning to get yourself going after a heavy drinking session?

(0) Never   (1) Less than monthly   (2) Monthly
(3) Weekly   (4) Daily or almost daily

7. How often during the past year have you had a feeling of guilt or
remorse after drinking?

(0) Never   (1) Less than monthly   (2) Monthly
(3) Weekly   (4) Daily or almost daily

8. How often during the past year have you been unable to remember
what happened the night before because you had been drinking?

(0) Never   (1) Less than monthly   (2) Monthly
(3) Weekly   (4) Daily or almost daily

---

[a] In determining the response categories, it has been assumed that one 'drink' contains 10 g alcohol.
In countries where the alcohol content of a standard drink differs by more than 25% from 10 g, the
response category should be modified accordingly.

9. Have you or someone else been injured as a result of your drinking?

(0) No   (1) Yes, but not in the last year

(4) Yes, during the last year

10. Has a relative or friend or a doctor or other health worker been
     concerned about your drinking or suggested you cut down?

(0) No   (1) Yes, but not in the last year

(4) Yes, during the last year

Addenbrooke's Cognitive Examination and Abbreviated Mental Test Scoring

Name   :

Date of birth :

Reference no. :

Years of education : _____

Date of testing   : __ / __ / __

Tester's name   : _____

All instructions to the tester are in italics. All instructions to be said aloud to the patient are in bold non-italic print.

ORIENTATION

Ask the subject the following questions and score a point for each correct answer. Record all errors.

Q1a) **What is the Year** _____
Season _____
Date* _____
Day _____
Month _____

*Allow an error of ± 2

Q1b) **Where are we Country** _____
County/State _____
Town _____
Hospital/building _____
Floor/Level* _____

Total score for orientation   [Score 0–10]

ATTENTION/CONCENTRATION

Q2) *Tell the subject I am going to ask you to recall the names of three things.*
Say aloud: **lemon, key, ball**. *Then ask the subject to repeat them. Give one point for each correct answer at first attempt only.*
If score <3 repeat all three items until the subject learns them all

Maximum trials allowed = 5.

[0–3]

Q3) *Ask the subject to* **take away 7 from 100.**
1. *Give one point only for the right answer* (93).
2. *If the subject's answer is wrong then tell the correct answer.*
3. *Ask the subject to* **now take away 7** *from the correct answer* (**93**).
Repeat steps 1 to 3 for a total of 5 subtractions (93, 86, 79, 72, 65). *Score the total number of correct subtractions.*
If score <5 then ask the subject to Spell '**WORLD**' **backwards.** *Score the number of letters in the correct order, eg dlorw = 4.*
Take score of better of the two tasks. Record errors:

[0–5]

Reproduced with permission from P.S. Mathuranath, et al., A brief cognitive test battery to differentiate Alzheimer's disease and frontotemporal dementia. Neurology. December 12, 2000 vol. 55 no. 11 1613–1620. © 2013 American Academy of Neurology.

MEMORY

Q4) *Ask the subject to recall the names of the 3 things learned earlier in question 2.*

Score one point for each correct answer. [0–3]

Q5) *Anterograde Memory: Tell the subject* **I will read a name and address and ask you to repeat it when I have finished.** *Now read aloud the following name and address. Score one point for each element recalled correctly. Regardless of the score after the first trial, repeat the instruction and the task twice in exactly the same way. Record scores for each of the three trials.*

	1st trial	2nd	3rd	5 min delay
Peter Marshall	—/—	—/—	—/—	—/—
42 Market Street	—/—	—/—	—/—	—/—
Chelmsford	—	—	—	—
Essex	/7	/7	/7	/7

Trial 1-3 [0–21]

5 min delay [0–7]

Q6) *Retrograde Memory: Score one point for each correct answer and record errors.* **Tell me the full name of**

the prime minister _____
the last prime minister _____
the Leader of the Opposition _____
the President of the United States of America _____ [0–4]

VERBAL FLUENCY

Q7) *Letter: Ask the subject to:* **tell me all the words you can think of, but not people and places, beginning with the letter P.** *Time the subject for 1 minute and record all answers in the space provided below. Error types: perseverations and intrusions.*

Q8) *Category: Say:* **Now tell me the names of as many animals as you can, beginning with any letter of the alphabet.** *Time the subject for 1 minute and record all responses in the space provided below. Error types: perseverations and intrusions.*

P

(start here) (continue) (continue)

_____

Animals

(start here) (continue)

_____

Raw Score		Scaled Score
P	Animal	
>17	>21	7
14–17	17–21	6
11–13	14–16	5
8–10	11–13	4
6–7	9–10	3
4–5	7–8	2
<4	<7	1

Record the total number of responses. To calculate the raw score give one point for each correct response and exclude all repetitions. Enter the scaled scores using the table shown above.

P : Total response _____ Raw score _____ Scaled Score [0–7] = _____

Animals : Total response _____ Raw score _____ Scaled Score [0–7] = _____

Total Scaled Score [0–14] _____

☐

LANGUAGE

Q9) *Naming: Show the subject the following two line-drawings and ask him/her to name each of them. Record responses and errors. Give one point for each correct response.*

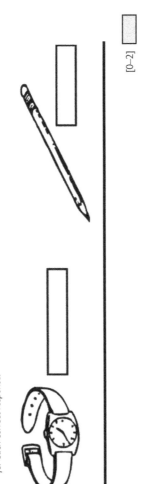

[0–2]

Q10) Naming: Show the subject the following ten line-drawings and ask him/her to name each of them. Record responses and errors. Give one point for each correct response. Allow close synonyms (e.g. tub for barrel; coronet for crown; dromedary for camel etc.)

[0–10]

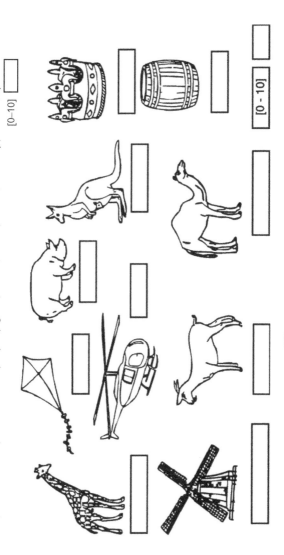

[0 – 10]

Q11) *Comprehension (one-stage):* Ask the subject to **please obey the following simple commands.**

- **point to the door**
- **point to the ceiling**

Show the subject the following instruction and ask him/her to **read this aloud and obey it.**

CLOSE YOUR EYES

[0–2]

Score one point if performed correctly.

[0–1]

Q12) *Comprehension (3-stages):* Give the subject a piece of paper and tell him to **take this paper in your hands. Fold it in half. Then put the paper on the floor.**

Score one point for each correctly performed step.

[0–3]

Q13) *Comprehension (complex grammar):* Ask the subject to **please obey the following commands.**

- **point to the ceiling then the door**
- **point to the door after touching the bed/desk**

Score one point for each correctly performed command.

[0–2]

Q14) *Repetition (single words):* Ask the subject to **repeat each of these words after me.** Score one point for each correct repetition. Allow only one repetition.

- **brown**
- **conversation**
- **articulate**

[0–3]

Q15) *Repetition (phrases): Ask the subject to repeat each of these phrases after me. Allow only one repetition.*
- No ifs, ands, or buts   [0–1]
- The orchestra played and the audience applauded   [0–1]

Q16) *Reading (regular): Ask the subject to read each of these words aloud and show him/her the following five words.*
- shed
- wipe
- board
- flame
- bridge

Score one point only if all five words are read correct.   [0–1]

Q17) *Reading (irregular): Ask the subject to read each of these words aloud and show him/her the following five words.*
- sew
- pint
- soot
- dough
- height

Score one point only if all five words are read correct.   [0–1]

Q18) *Writing:* Ask the subject to **make up a sentence and write it down in the space below.** *If stuck suggest a topic e.g. weather, journey. Score one point if the sentence has a correct subject and verb and is meaningful.*

_____

_____

[0–1]

Q19) *Now to check delayed recall ask the subject* **Can you tell me the name and address that I told you and that you practised at the beginning of the test.** *Record points, scores and errors as for question 5 in the space provided in question 5.*

VISUOSPATIAL ABILITIES

Q20) *Overlapping pentagons:* Show the subject the following figure and ask him/her to **copy this diagram in the space provided next to it.**

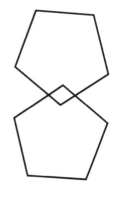

[0–1]

Score one point if copied correct.

Q21) Wire cube: Show the subject the following figure and ask him/her to copy this diagram in the space provided next to it.

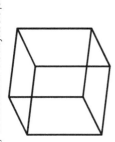

[0–1]

Score one point if copied correct.

Q22) *Clock:* Ask the subject to draw a clock-face with numbers and the hands at ten past five.

[0–3] ☐

Score one point each, for correct circle, numbering of the clock-face and position of the hands.

<u>CHECK:</u> Have you tested and recorded the delayed recall for name and address in Q5?

OVERALL SCORES

MMSE**	=	/30
ACE*	=	/100

*Sum of scores entered in the shaded boxes. *Sum of scores entered in all boxes.

**Sum of scores entered in all boxes.

Abbreviated mental test scoring

1. Age (must be correct to score).
2. Time (to nearest hour).
3. Now give them an address for recall (3 items only—e.g. 98, Primrose Hill, Wimbledon—*repeated by the patient to ensure that it has been heard correctly*—don't score yet).
4. Year (must be correct).
5. Where are we?
6. Recognition of two people (usually the doctor and the carer).
7. Date of birth (they must give date, month, and year to score).
8. Year of world war (must be correct year of starting and stopping).
9. Name of present monarch.
10. Count backwards from 20 to 1 (each number from 20 back to 1 has to be in order—one missed number: no score).

Now ask them to recall the address given as point 3 above (2+ items recalled scores the point).

Scoring is one mark for each exactly correct. (Scoring is generally accepted as 6 or below as indicating probable dementia. However a score of 7 or 8 should be treated with caution and repeated.)

Hodkinson M (1972). Evaluation of a mental test score for assessment of mental impairment in the elderly, *Age and Ageing*, 1, 233–8, by permission of Oxford University Press.

The 'SAD PERSONS' scale

Table A3.1 The 'SAD PERSONS' scale

S	Sex is male
A	Age is older than 45 or younger than 19 years
D	Depression
P	Previous attempts
E	Ethanol abuse
R	Rational thinking loss (particularly psychosis)
S	Social support is lacking
O	Organized plan
N	No spouse
S	Sickness (physical illness, especially if painful)

Each positive item receives a score of 1. A flexible use of the following evaluation can be helpful:

- Score 0–2: Low risk. Discharge and outpatient follow-up.
- Score 3–4: Moderate risk. Close monitoring as outpatient. Consider admission.
- Score 5–6: High risk. Admission is advised, especially if support from environment seems uncertain.
- Score 7–10: Very high risk of suicide. Admission required.

This article was published in Psychosomatics, Volume 24, Issue 4, William M. Patterson, Henry H. Dohn, Julian Bird, et al. Evaluation of suicidal patients: The SAD PERSONS scale, pp343–345, 348–349, Copyright Elsevier (1983). Reproduced with permission.

Alcohol Withdrawal Assessment Scoring Guidelines (CIWA-Ar)

Nausea/Vomiting - Rate on scale 0 - 7.
0 - none
1 - mild nausea with no vomiting
2
3

4 - intermittent nausea
5
6

7 - constant nausea and frequent dry heaves and vomiting

Tremors - have patient extend arms & spread fingers. Rate on scale 0 - 7.
0 - no tremor
1 - not visible, but can be felt fingertip to fingertip
2
3
4 - moderate, with patient's arms extended
5
6
7 - severe, even w/ arms not extended

Anxiety - Rate on scale 0 - 7.
0 - no anxiety, patient at ease
1 - mildly anxious
2
3
4 - moderately anxious or guarded, so anxiety is inferred
5
6
7 - equivalent to acute panic states seen in severe delirium or acute schizophrenic reactions.

Agitation - Rate on scale 0 - 7.
0 - normal activity
1 - somewhat normal activity
2
3
4 - moderately fidgety and restless
5
6
7 - paces back and forth, or constantly thrashes about

Paroxysmal Sweats - Rate on Scale 0 - 7.
0 - no sweats
1 - barely perceptible sweating, palms moist
2
3
4 - beads of sweat obvious on forehead
5
6

7 - drenching sweats

Orientation and clouding of sensorium - Ask, "What day is this? Where are you? Who am I?" Rate scale 0 - 4.
0 - oriented

1 - cannot do serial additions or is uncertain about date

2 - disoriented to date by no more than 2 calendar days

3 - disoriented to date by more than 2 calendar days

4 - disoriented to place and / or person

Tactile disturbances - Ask, "Have you experienced any itching, pins & needles sensation, burning or numbness, or a feeling of bugs crawling on or under your skin?"

0 - none
1 - very mild itching, pins & needles, burning, or numbness
2 - mild itching, pins & needles, burning, or numbness
3 - moderate itching, pins & needles, burning, or numbness
4 - moderate hallucinations
5 - severe hallucinations
6 - extremely severe hallucinations
7 - continuous hallucinations

Auditory Disturbances - Ask, "Are you more aware of sounds around you? Are they harsh? Do they startle you? Do you hear anything that disturbs you or that you know isn't there?"

0 - not present
1 - Very mild harshness or ability to startle
2 - mild harshness or ability to startle
3 - moderate harshness or ability to startle
4 - moderate hallucinations
5 - severe hallucinations
6 - extremely severe hallucinations
7 - continuous hallucinations

Visual disturbances - Ask, "Does the light appear to be too bright? Is its color different than normal? Does it hurt your eyes? Are you seeing anything that disturbs you or that you know isn't there?"

0 - not present
1 - very mild sensitivity
2 - mild sensitivity
3 - moderate sensitivity
4 - moderate hallucinations
5 - severe hallucinations
6 - extremely severe hallucinations
7 - continuous hallucinations

Headache - Ask, "Does your head feel different than usual? Does it feel like there is a band around your head?" Do not rate dizziness or lightheadedness.

0 - not present
1 - very mild
2 - mild
3 - moderate
4 - moderately severe
5 - severe
6 - very severe
7 - extremely severe

Procedure:
1. Assess and rate each of the 10 criteria of the CIWA scale. Add up the scores for all ten criteria. This is the total CIWA-Ar score for the patient at that time.
2. If < 10 additional medication not required. > 15 is considered severe withdrawal.

Antipsychotic depot injections: suggested adult doses and frequencies

Typical antipsychotics

Drug	Trade name	Test dose (mg)	Dose range (mg/week)	Dosing interval (weeks)	Comments
Flupentixol decanoate	Depixol®	20	12.5–400	2–4	Mood elevating; may worsen agitation
Fluphenazine decanoate	Modecate®	12.5	6.25–50	2–5	Avoid in depression, high EPSE
Haloperidol decanoate	Haldol Decanoate®	25[a]	12.5–75	4	High EPSE, low incidence of sedation
Pipotiazine palmitate	Piportil Depot®	25	12.5–50	4	Lower incidence of EPSE
Zuclopenthixol decanoate	Clopixol®	100	100–600	2–4	Useful in agitation and aggression

EPSE, extrapyramidal side effects.

[a] Test dose not stated by manufacturer.

Notes

• Give a quarter or half stated doses in elderly.

• After test dose, wait 4–10 days before starting titration to maintenance therapy.

• Dose range is given in mg/week for convenience only; avoid using shorter dose intervals than those recommended except in exceptional circumstances (e.g. long interval necessitates high-volume (>3–4 ml) injection).

Atypical antipsychotics

Drug	Trade name	Test dose (mg)	Dose range (mg/week)	Dosing interval (weeks)	Comments
Risperidone microspheres	Risperdal Consta®	Not required	12.5–25	2	Lower incidence of EPSE
Paliperidone palmitate	Xeplion®	Not required	6.25–37.5	4	Lower incidence of EPSE
Olanzapine embonate	ZypAdhera®	Not required	75–150	2–4	Risk of post injection syndrome (delirium) requires clinical observation for 3 hours after administration.
Aripiprazole (powder and solvent)	Abilify Maintena®	Not required	50–100	4	Lower incidence of metabolic syndrome and no effect on prolactin.

Notes

- 25–50 mg every 2 weeks of risperidone long-acting injection (RLAI) appears to be as effective as oral doses of 2–6 mg/day.
- Prior testing of tolerability with oral risperidone is desirable but not always practical.
- RLAI takes 3–4 weeks for the first injection to reach therapeutic plasma levels requiring cover (e.g. oral risperidone) for at least 3 weeks and then tapering over 1–2 weeks.
- Switching from typical depot to RLAI: give the first injection of RLAI 1 week *before* the last typical depot is given.
- Paliperidone is a major active metabolite of risperidone but the depot preparation reaches therapeutic plasma levels in approximately a day making cover, in theory, not required.
- Patients need to have demonstrated response and tolerability to oral aripiprazole before depot. Watch for insomnia and akathisia.
- Oral aripiprazole 10–20 mg should be continued for 14 days after first aripiprazole injection or if given after 5–6 week interval.
- 400 mg IM every 4 weeks is typical starting dose of aripiprazole. It can be reduced to 300 mg or (rarely) 200 mg.

Appendix 6

Equivalent doses, maximum daily doses, and adverse effects of antipsychotics

Equivalent doses of typical antipsychotics

Drug	Equivalent dose (consensus)	Range of values in literature (mg/day)
Chlorpromazine	100 mg/day	–
Fluphenazine	2 mg/day	2–5 mg/day
Trifluoperazine	5 mg/day	2.5–5 mg/day
Flupentixol	3 mg/day	2–3 mg/day
Zuclopenthixol	25 mg/day	25–60 mg/day
Haloperidol	3 mg/day	1.5–5 mg/day
Sulpiride	200 mg/day	200–270 mg/day
Fluphenazine depot	5 mg/week	1–12.5 mg/week
Pipotiazine depot	10 mg/week	10–12.5 mg/week
Flupentixol depot	10 mg/week	10–20 mg/week
Zuclopenthixol depot	100 mg/week	40–100 mg/week
Haloperidol depot	15 mg/week	5–25 mg/week

All values should be regarded as approximate.

No equivalent doses are given for atypical antipsychotics because their more variable D2 occupancy makes this illogical.

Oral/parenteral dose equivalents

Drug	Oral dose (mg)	Equivalent i.m. or i.v. dose (mg)
Benzodiazepines		
Diazepam	10	10
Lorazepam	4	4
Antipsychotics		
Chlorpromazine	100	25–50
Haloperidol	10	5
Promazine	200	200
Anticholinergics		
Procyclidine	10	7.5

Note

Because of the variation in bioavailability with some drugs, prescriptions should always specify the dose *and* a single route of administration.

Maximum daily doses of oral antipsychotics

Drug	Licensed maximum dose
Chlorpromazine	1000 mg/day
Trifluoperazine	None
Haloperidol	30 mg/day
Sulpiride	2400 mg/day
Clozapine	900 mg/day (anticonvulsant cover for doses over 600 mg)
Risperidone	16 mg/day
Paliperidone	12 mg/day
Amisulpride	1200 mg/day
Olanzapine	20 mg/day
Quetiapine	750–800 mg/day
Aripiprazole	30 mg/day

Note

Doses above these maxima should only be used in extreme circumstances; there is no evidence for improved efficacy. Always follow Royal College of Psychiatrists guidelines.

Beware that plasma levels can be increased with smoking cessation and drug interactions.

Relative adverse effects of antipsychotics

Drug	Sedation	Extrapyramidal	Anticholinergic	Hypotension	Prolactin elevation	Weight gain	Diabetes
Chlorpromazine	+++	++	++	+++	+++	++	++
Fluphenazine	+	+++	++	+	+++	+	+
Trifluoperazine	+	+++	+/-	+	+++	+	+/-
Flupentixol	+	++	++	+	+++	++	+
Pipothiazine	++	++	++	++	+++	++	+
Zuclopenthixol	++	++	++	+	+++	++	+
Haloperidol	+	+++	+	+	+++	+	+/-
Sulpiride	-	+	-	-	+++	+	+
Clozapine	+++	-	+++	+++	-	+++	+++
Risperidone[a]	+	+	+	++	+++	++	+
Paliperidone	+	+	+	++	+++	++	+
Olanzapine	++	+/-	+	+	+	+++	+++
Quetiapine	++	-	+	++	-	++	++
Amisulpride	-	+	-	-	+++	-	+
Aripiprazole	-	+/-	-	-	-	+/-	+

+++ High incidence/severity; ++ moderate; + low; -, very low/none.
[a] Akathisia common with risperidone.

Clozapine: management of adverse effects

Table A7.1 Clozapine: management of adverse effects

Adverse effect	Time course	Action
Sedation	First 4 weeks. May persist, but usually wears off	Give smaller dose in the mornings. Some patients can only cope with single night-time dosing. Reduce dose if necessary
Hypersalivation	First 4 weeks. May persist, but usually wears off. Often very troublesome at night	Give hyoscine 300 micrograms (Kwells) chewed and swallowed at night. Propantheline 15 mg tds may be used but worsens anticholinergic effects. Pirenzepine may be tried. Patients do not always mind excess salivation—treatment not always required
Constipation	Usually persists	Recommend high-fibre diet. Bulk-forming laxatives ± stimulants may be used
Hypotension	First 4 weeks	Advise patient to take time when standing up. Reduce dose or slow down rate of increase. If severe, consider moclobemide and Bovril
Tachycardia	First 4 weeks, but often persists	Often occurs if dose escalation is too rapid. Inform patient that it is not dangerous. Give small dose of beta-blocker if necessary
Weight gain	Usually during the first year of treatment	Dietary counselling is essential. Advice may be more effective if given before weight gain occurs. Weight gain is common and often profound (>2 stones)
Fever	First 3 weeks	Give antipyretic. NB: This fever is not usually related to blood dyscrasias
Seizures	May occur at any time	Dose related. Consider prophylactic valproate[a] if on high dose. After a seizure withhold clozapine for 1 day. Restart at reduced dose. Give sodium valproate
Nausea	First 6 weeks	May give antiemetic. Avoid prochlorperazine and metoclopramide (EPSE)
Myocarditis[b]	First 8 weeks	Eosinophilia, raised CRP, CK, and troponin aid diagnosis. Stop clozapine and cardiology follow-up
Neutropenia/ agranulocytosis	First 18 weeks (but may occur at any time)	Stop clozapine; WCC monitoring
Nocturnal enuresis	May occur at any time	Try manipulating dose schedule. Avoid fluids before bedtime. In severe cases, desmopressin is usually effective.

[a] Usual dose is 1000–2000 mg/day. Plasma levels may be useful as a rough guide to dosing— aim for 50–100 mg/L. Use of modified-release preparation (Epilim Chrono®) may aid compliance: can be given once daily and may be better tolerated.

[b] Consider myocarditis with symptoms of chest pain, dyspnea, tachycardia at rest, palpitations, arrhythmia or other ECG abnormalities, flu-like symptoms, signs of heart failure.

Index